Children and Emotion

Contributions to Human Development

Vol. 26

Series Editor

Larry Nucci Berkeley, Calif.

Children and Emotion

New Insights into Developmental Affective Science

Volume Editor

Kristin Hansen Lagattuta Davis, Calif.

1 figure, 2014

KARGER

Basel · Freiburg · Paris · London · New York · New Delhi · Bangkok · Beijing · Tokyo · Kuala Lumpur · Singapore · Sydney

Kristin Hansen Lagattuta
Department of Psychology and
Center for Mind and Brain
University of California, Davis
1 Shields Avenue
Davis, CA 95616, USA

Library of Congress Cataloging-in-Publication Data

Children and emotion : new insights into developmental affective science / volume editor, Kristin Hansen Lagattuta.
pages cm. -- (Contributions to human development, ISSN 0301-4193 ; vol. 26)
Includes bibliographical references and index.
ISBN 978-3-318-02488-3 (soft cover : alk. paper) -- ISBN 978-3-318-02489-0 (electronic version) 1. Emotions in children I. Lagattuta, Kristin Hansen.
BF723.E6C46 2014
155.4'124--dc23
2013033894

Bibliographic Indices. This publication is listed in bibliographic services, including Current Contents®.

www.karger.com
Printed in Germany on acid-free and non-aging paper (ISO 9706) by Kraft Druck GmbH, Ettlingen
ISSN 0301–4193
e-ISSN 1664–2570
ISBN 978–3–318–02488–3
e-ISBN 978–3–318–02489–0

Dedicated to
Kaitlyn, John, and Sarah

Contents

Introduction: Integrated Approaches to Studying the Development of Emotion

Kristin Hansen Lagattuta

Department of Psychology and Center for Mind and Brain, University of California, Davis, Calif., USA

Emotions are central to everyday human lives and relationships. How we attend to, interpret, talk about and respond to emotional displays of others, regulate our own internal feelings, reminisce about emotions from the past, and anticipate our future affective reactions critically influences our well-being and decision making, including how we form, maintain, and confront challenges in social relationships. For these reasons, developmental scientists have focused strong research attention on the development of emotion processing, understanding, and regulation in infancy and childhood, including sources of individual differences (e.g. genetics, biology, family, culture, early experience). A basic search in July 2013 on the PsycINFO behavioral sciences database for 'children and emotion' yielded 18,649 entries, 'development and emotion' 22,971, and 'emotional development' 53,280 – with all categories showing rapid growth in publication numbers over the past 10 years. Indeed, for all three searches, more than 50% of the total scholarly works were published within the past decade alone.

The chapters in this volume summarize and critically evaluate cutting-edge research on children and emotion. In selecting topics and authors for this book, I aimed to incorporate leaders and rising stars in the field who, as a group, use multiple levels of analysis (behavioral, cognitive, social, neural, genetic) and diverse research methods (e.g. observational studies, experimental studies, narrative analyses, self-report measures, parent-report measures, eye-tracking, heart rate, cortisol, ERP, fMRI). Together, the nine chapters cover age-related changes and individual variability in infants' and children's attention, processing, understanding, conversation, regulation, and expression of emotions in typical and atypical populations, including connections to parenting and wider cultural values and norms. Due to the centrality of emotions to children's (and adults') lives and experiences, this book will be useful to researchers, educators, parents, and policy makers. Below, I highlight the key features of each contribution.

In the first chapter, Hoehl critically reviews behavioral (preferential looking, habituation, eye-tracking) and neurophysiological research (ERP studies) on how infants attend to, process, and discriminate facial emotion expressions during the first year of life. Of central focus is the development of attentional biases towards negative emotions (especially anger and fear), including variations in attention (e.g., to negative vs. positive emotion faces, to eye vs. mouth regions) based on whether the person expressing the emotion is looking directly ahead or at a specific referent. She further explores how variability in infant temperament, genetics, parenting, and experience shape how infants process and respond to emotion signals. Hoehl ends by urging researchers to integrate multiple technologies and levels of analysis (e.g., eye tracking, neurophysiological measures, behavior) to advance the science of infant emotion processing.

The second chapter, by Hastings, Kahle and Han, explores the benefits and complexities of incorporating assessments of biological activity into developmental emotion research. Developmental scientists are more frequently relying on psychophysiological techniques (e.g., neurophysiological, neuroendocrinological, autonomic, electromyographic measures) to understand how children regulate their emotions, as well as how children use emotion to regulate cognition and behavior. As Hastings and colleagues aptly argue, this research enterprise poses a significant challenge because 'physiological systems are developing, emotions are developing, and the relations between physiology and emotions also are developing'. As with Hoehl's chapter, Hastings and colleagues further discuss sources of individual differences in relation to temperament, genetics, parenting, and early experience, and they provide ideas for future work.

Examination of atypical life experiences and maladaptive developmental patterns can help elucidate the mechanisms of normal development. Thus, in the third chapter, Cicchetti and Ng investigate the impact of physical maltreatment on how young children perceive, regulate, process, express, and understand emotions. The authors argue that deviations in all of these areas begin during infancy, with these perturbations both reflecting and strengthening the abnormal development of emotion-related neural networks. Converging evidence from behavioral and neuroscience approaches support these interpretations, especially regarding relations between abusive home environments and the development of hypervigilance to anger. In addition to giving multiple suggestions for future research, Cicchetti and Ng further address how scientific inquiry can inform the design of effective interventions.

Pérez-Edgar, Taber-Thomas, Auday and Morales continue this discussion of atypical emotional development in their chapter by exploring the emergence of childhood anxiety. They argue that although temperament is a significant risk factor for developing anxiety (especially behavioral inhibition or temperamental shyness), children's attention biases to threat-related information modulate this link between temperament and anxiety. Pérez-Edgar and colleagues draw from behavioral (e.g., dot-probe tasks), psychophysiological (e.g., eye tracking) and neuroscience research (ERP, fMRI) to substantiate this temperament-attention-anxiety network. They further describe how training programs aimed at modifying attention biases provide a promising approach for both preventing and reducing anxiety symptoms in children and adults.

In the fifth chapter, Lemerise and Harper shift emphasis towards how children develop emotional competence in the context of family and peer relationships. Multiple studies converge to indicate that warm and supportive parent-child relationships provide an essential foundation for children to develop skills at identifying, understanding, regulating, talking about, and responding to their own and others' emotions. Moreover, individual differences in emotional competence predict children's concurrent and future peer relations and behavioral adjustment. The authors close with arguing that intervention programs designed to improve preschoolers' emotion knowledge and emotion regulatory skills can help reduce socio-emotional problems and academic difficulties in the critical transition to school.

Because emotion researchers have concentrated primarily on Western populations, the literature provides an imbalanced perspective on emotional development. Thus, in the chapter by Camras, Shuster, and Fraumeni, they take a cross-cultural approach when considering relations between parents' beliefs, attitudes, and values, their parenting practices, and children's emotional competence. They use numerous research examples to highlight how the same emotions can be interpreted, valued, or expressed in different ways in different cultures. Moreover, the same parenting behaviors can be motivated by different beliefs about emotions and predict different child outcomes. The authors end with strategies for building research collaborations with non-Western nations; partnerships essential for constructing comprehensive theories of emotion.

Next, Fivush delves deeper into one of the central ways in which children learn about emotions – through parentally guided conversations about past emotional experiences. Using sociocultural and feminist theories to frame her arguments, Fivush proposes that through parent-child reminiscing about the past children develop an autobiographical voice that reflects their understanding of their own and others' emotional lives. Cross-sectional and longitudinal studies in childhood and adolescence reveal significant differences in how mothers versus fathers discuss emotions as well as how parents talk about emotions with sons versus daughters. In turn, these co-constructed narratives shape how children learn to interpret, express, and regulate emotions appropriate for their social, historical, and cultural place.

The next chapter expands this focus on family conversation to investigate how parent-child conversations about internal mental states more broadly – about emotions, thoughts, and desires – not only relate to children's growing emotion knowledge but also to their understanding of their own and others' psychological lives (theory of mind). Hughes, White and Ensor critically review a broad base of literature demonstrating how children's linguistic environments, especially parent-child talk about emotions and the mind, causally shape their social-cognitive development. They consider not only typically developing children in Western samples, but also children with deafness, children diagnosed with autism, and children from non-Western cultural communities. Training and intervention studies help to elucidate further the mechanisms by which parent-child conversations impact children's learning about the social world.

In the final chapter, Harris, de Rosnay and Ronfard provide a thoughtful analysis of an intriguing paradoxical pattern in young children's understanding of emotions – a lag between their understanding that a person can have a mistaken (or false) belief and their ability to infer the person's emotions based on this belief. For example, whereas 4- to 6-year-olds frequently state that Little Red Riding Hood thinks her grandmother is lying in the bed (as opposed to a disguised, threatening wolf) they nevertheless predict that she will feel afraid (because it really is the wolf). That is, when children forecast emotions, the reality of the situation often trumps what they know about belief. The authors evaluate several alternative explanations for this disconnect between children's belief and emotion judgments, and they suggest avenues for future research on developmental changes and individual differences in children's emotion understanding.

This book project would not have taken off without the enthusiastic participation of this elite group of researchers. I am extremely grateful for their informative, thought-provoking, and research-inspiring chapters. I greatly admire their methodological rigor and creative approaches to examining emotion from the lens of development. I also wish to thank Larry Nucci, the editor of this volume series, for giving me this opportunity, the editorial staff at Karger for their assistance with the production and promotion of the book (especially Sandra Braun, Brigitte Thierstein, and Angela Gasser), my graduate and undergraduate students who helped in the editing process (especially Hannah Kramer), and my husband and three children for providing continued support and multiple opportunities to learn first-hand about emotion in the lives of children and families.

Hansen Lagattuta K (ed): Children and Emotion. New Insights into Developmental Affective Sciences.
Contrib Hum Dev. Basel, Karger, 2014, vol 26, pp 1–12 (DOI: 10.1159/000354346)

Emotion Processing in Infancy

Stefanie Hoehl
Institute of Psychology, Heidelberg University, Heidelberg, Germany

Abstract

This chapter provides an overview of behavioral and neurophysiological research on the discrimination and categorization of emotional expressions in the first year of life. Three recent lines of research with theoretical implications beyond perceptual discrimination of facial expressions are discussed. The first focuses on the development of attentional biases towards facial expressions. Between 5 and 7 months of age infants start to attend preferentially towards fearful faces rather than happy faces and disengage attention less easily from fearful faces than from happy or neutral faces. Recent studies have shown that there are individual differences between infants regarding these biases, which may potentially be informative with respect to later emotion regulation abilities or affective dysfunctions. Studies within the second line of research have shown that infants process emotional facial expressions differently depending on the referent of the expression. For instance, 7-month-olds respond with increased attention to a fearful face that looks towards an object than a fearful face without a clear referent. In contrast, an angry face with eyes gazing straight ahead receives more attention by infants of the same age than an angry face looking to the side. This research and its implications on the development of social referencing and observational fear learning will also be discussed. In the third line of research, eye tracking is used to examine infants' looking patterns at faces with different emotional expressions. I will conclude with open questions and future directions for the field.

Emotional facial expressions are powerful means to communicate affective states as well as information about the environment, such as potential threats emanating from an object or a person [Hooker, Germine, Knight & D'Esposito, 2006; Vuilleumier, 2005]. They can further aid in predicting the behavior of people; for example, anger can be accompanied by forceful action, making the detection of this emotion important for children with abusive caregivers [Pollak, Cicchetti, Hornung & Reed, 2000]. Developmental psychology research has shown that preverbal infants are well able to perceptually discriminate emotional facial expressions from early on in development and start to categorize facial expressions within the first 6 months after birth [Leppänen & Nelson, 2009]. This research, which will be briefly summarized below, has been mainly conducted using classic behavioral paradigms like preferential looking and habituation techniques. Questions still remain, however, regarding when infants start to understand the meanings of different emotional expressions.

Only recently have researchers begun to use neurophysiological measures and eye tracking to look more closely at how different emotional expressions are processed and how infants' attention towards objects is affected by emotional facial expressions [Hoehl, Wiese & Striano, 2008; Hunnius, de Wit, Vrins & von Hofsten, 2011]. Furthermore, individual differences regarding attentional biases towards facial expressions are now increasingly explored, which may provide information on later emotion regulation abilities and affective dysfunctions [Leppänen et al., 2011; see also Perez-Edgar, this vol.]. I will review these new lines of research and conclude with a discussion of open questions and potential future directions of research. In this chapter, I focus on facial expressions of emotions. For reviews on infants' emotion processing in the auditory domain and studies using multimodal stimuli see Walker-Andrews [1997] and Hoehl [2008]. The neural networks involved in the development of emotion processing have been recently reviewed by Leppänen and Nelson [2009].

Discrimination and Categorization of Emotional Facial Expressions in Infancy

In classic studies on the discrimination of facial emotional expressions infants have usually been tested using preferential looking and/or habituation paradigms [see de Haan & Nelson, 1998, for a review]. Preferential looking paradigms measure spontaneous looking preferences for certain visual stimuli over others. In habituation studies, one stimulus (e.g., an emotional face) is presented repeatedly until infants lose interest and cease looking (i.e., until they habituate). Then a new picture (e.g., a face with a different expression) is shown. If infants detect the difference between the familiar and the new stimulus they typically show recovery of attention and increased interest in the new picture. Using habituation techniques it is also possible to examine categorization of emotional expressions by showing different individual faces with the same emotional expression during the habituation phase and a new person with a different expression during test. Using behavioral methods such as these, researchers have shown that infants who are only a few days old look longer at a happy face than at a fearful face [Farroni, Menon, Rigato & Johnson, 2007]. By 3 months of age infants discriminate smiling faces from frowning and surprised faces [Barrera & Maurer, 1981; Young-Browne, Rosenfeld & Horowitz, 1977]. Furthermore, 4- and 7-month-olds prefer to look at happy faces over angry and neutral faces [Grossmann, Striano & Friederici, 2007; LaBarbera, Izard, Vietze & Parisi, 1976; Wilcox & Clayton, 1968].

Young infants' early discrimination and visual preference for happy faces over other expressions may result from their predominantly positive interactions with adults in the first days and months after birth [Vaish, Grossmann & Woodward, 2008]. Negative emotional expressions, in contrast, may become relevant to infants only when they start to crawl or walk. Improvements in infants' self-locomotive abilities increase the risk of harm in novel or dangerous situations, prompting caregivers to express negative affect more frequently to control infants' behavior. Infants, in turn, need to learn how to adjust their actions according to these emotional signals and reactions [Campos et al., 2000]. By 7 months, around the age they typically start to locomote, infants are able to discriminate most basic emotional facial expressions, including negative emotions like fear and anger, and they are also able to categorize several facial emotional expressions [de Haan & Nelson, 1998; Leppänen & Nelson, 2006, 2009].

Experiences in early development seem to have considerable influence on facial emotion processing. For instance, physically abused 3- to 5-year-olds are overly sensitive to expressions of anger and show a response bias towards anger when matching facial expressions to the emotions of the protagonist of a story [Pollak et al., 2000]. Neurophysiological studies also point to altered emotion processing in maltreated children at 30 months [Cicchetti & Curtis, 2005] and at 6–12 years of age [Pollak, Klorman, Thatcher & Cicchetti, 2001]. Notably, some of these children experienced maltreatment already in the first year of life. It is possible that the observed biases and processing differences develop very early. A study with 7- to 32-month-olds who were reared in institutionalized settings (i.e., Romanian orphanages) provides further evidence for early effects of adverse rearing environments on infants' and toddlers' brain responses by showing abnormalities in children's event-related potentials (ERP) to emotional expressions when compared to a control group of children who lived with their parents [Parker & Nelson, 2005; see also Cicchetti & Ng, this vol.; Pérez-Edgar, et al., this vol.].

Attention Biases for Emotional Faces: Individual Differences and Implications

One of the most robust findings regarding infant emotion processing is that by 7 months of age infants prefer to look at a fearful face rather than a happy face [de Haan, Belsky, Reid, Volein & Johnson, 2004; Kotsoni, de Haan & Johnson, 2001; Ludemann & Nelson, 1988; Nelson & Dolgin, 1985; Peltola, Leppänen, Maki & Hietanen, 2009]. Consistent with this behavioral finding, 7-month-olds respond with an increased amplitude of the Nc (negative central) component to fearful faces compared with happy faces in studies using ERP [Grossmann et al., 2011; Nelson & de Haan, 1996; Peltola, Leppänen, Maki, et al., 2009]. Amplitude of the Nc is typically taken as an index of the amount of attention directed at a visual stimulus [Reynolds & Richards, 2005; Richards, 2003]. Thus, infants consistently direct more attention towards fearful faces than happy faces. This attention bias emerges between 5 and 7 months of age both on the behavioral level and the neuronal level [Peltola, Leppänen, Maki, et al., 2009]. As mentioned above, infants younger than 7 months of age typically prefer to look at positive expressions rather than negative expressions in a range of behavioral paradigms [Leppänen & Nelson, 2006; Vaish et al., 2008].

What may be the function of this early developing attention bias towards fearful faces and what are the mechanisms of its development? Infants' preference for fearful faces may in part be due to the relative novelty of this expression. Before infants are able to crawl or walk they are typically rarely exposed to negative emotional expressions by their caregivers [Campos et al., 2000]. The development of infants' attention bias for fearful faces coincides with an expansion of their exploration of the environment resulting from increasing motor abilities. When independently moving around they encounter dangerous situations more often, and, consequently, they more frequently elicit negative emotional reactions in their caregivers [Campos et al., 2000]. That is, infants begin to attend to fearful faces around the time they start to encounter this expression more commonly in their daily interactions with caregivers who try to keep them from harm [Campos et al., 2000]. This speaks against a pure novelty preference interpretation of the fear-over-happiness bias. In addition, it is not clear why a novelty preference should not be present in 5-month-olds who have even less experience with this expression [Peltola, Leppänen, Maki, et al., 2009]. Furthermore, infants do not seem to preferentially attend to other types of unusual facial expressions, such as blowing cheeks [Peltola, Leppänen, Palokangas & Hietanen, 2008]. In contrast, infants' increased attention to fearful expressions coincides with the time they start to learn about their meaning. This process may be associated with neuronal development and maturation of fear-processing networks in the brain [Leppänen & Nelson, 2009].

Different laboratories have documented the described bias in many studies using behavioral and neurophysiological methods. This indicates that it may constitute a universal mechanism occurring around the same age in many if not all infants. However, two studies have found individual differences among infants regarding this bias. For instance, de Haan et al. [2004] looked at associations with maternal personality and infant temperament in 7-month-olds. Highly fearful infants showed an increased Nc for fearful compared with happy faces on the right hemisphere, whereas infants scoring low on temperamental fearfulness did not. In addition, maternal affect interacted with infant temperament in that highly positive infants (i.e., infants smiling and laughing a lot) with highly positive mothers showed a larger Nc for fearful than happy faces on both hemispheres, whereas no significant difference was found for the other groups [de Haan et al., 2004]. The authors conclude that both high familiarity with positive affect (and thus decreased sensitivity to this expression) and temperamental fearfulness (and thus increased reactions to novelty and/or the threat-related signal value of fearful faces) may contribute to the observed attention bias with partly different neuronal signatures for both factors. In this view, infants may need to acquire a certain amount of visual exposure to happy faces before they lose interest in them and start to prefer attending to the more novel fearful expressions [see also Vaish et al., 2008]. The lack of an effect of maternal negative affect in this study may result from limited variance in negative affect in this healthy sample.

More recently, Grossmann and colleagues looked at gene polymorphisms related to dopamine and serotonin activity in the brain and their effects on 7-month-olds' attention bias to fearful versus happy faces [Grossmann et al., 2011]. They found that variants of the *COMT* gene that affect dopamine concentration in prefrontal cortex are related to infants' neuronal responses to fearful faces. Variants of the *5-HTTLPR* that are associated with the serotonin system, in contrast, were related to infants' processing of positive facial expressions. Both genetic variants also correlated with infant temperament. These studies demonstrate that interesting individual differences can be found when investigating a phenomenon that seems to generally occur in infants around the same age. It should be noted, though, that cross-cultural studies on this topic are still lacking, leaving open, whether the phenomenon is universal or culture-related.

Another series of studies has explored attention biases to fearful faces using attention disengagement tasks rather than overall preferences in attention allocation towards different expressions [Peltola et al., 2008; Peltola, Leppänen, Vogel-Farley, Hietanen & Nelson, 2009]. In the gap/overlap task a central stimulus is presented on a screen. After a certain amount of time, a peripheral stimulus is presented either following disappearance of the central stimulus (gap trials) or simultaneously to the central stimulus (overlap trials). Measuring how often and how quickly infants shift gaze from the central position to the peripheral target allows for testing how effectively attention can be disengaged from different kinds of central stimuli. Furthermore, disengagement should be more difficult in overlap trials than in gap trials. Consistent with their hypothesis, Peltola and colleagues found that, in overlap trials, 7-month-old infants maintained fixation on the central stimulus more often when it was a fearful face as compared to a happy face or matched visual noise [Peltola et al., 2008]. That is, they more often failed to direct attention away from a fearful face than from a happy face or a non-face. This finding was extended in another experiment [Peltola, Leppänen, Vogel-Farley, et al., 2009]. In this study 7-month-olds took longer to disengage attention from a centrally presented fearful face than from a happy or a neutral face or a neutral face with fearful eyes. The latter finding also implicates that wide-opened eyes as a prominent feature of fearful faces do not account for infants' attention bias to fearful faces alone.

Using the same paradigm, Leppänen and colleagues have also examined individual differences in infants' ability to disengage attention from emotionally salient stimuli [Leppänen et al., 2011]. Overall, 7-month-olds in this study had the greatest difficulties at disengaging attention from a centrally presented fearful face as compared to a happy or neutral face or a matched visual noise stimulus. In addition, the authors report a significantly greater number of missed saccades (i.e., infants kept fixating on the central stimulus) for carriers of the T allele compared to G/G homozygotes of the *TPH2* gene which has been related to serotonin concentrations in the brain [Leppänen et al., 2011]. This effect was particularly strong in trials with emotionally significant faces (happy and fearful) as central stimuli. Furthermore, through its influence on attention disengagement as a means of emotion regulation, the *TPH2* seems to be linked with infants' temperamental soothability as reported by their parents [Leppänen et al., 2011].

In summary, the studies reviewed in this section have shown that by 7 months of age infants preferentially attend to fearful more than happy faces. Furthermore, infants at this age have greater difficulties disengaging attention from a centrally presented fearful face compared to other face or non-face stimuli to shift gaze towards a peripheral target. The functional significance and developmental mechanisms of these biases are not yet fully understood. Relating individual differences in these attention biases to gene polymorphisms and other factors, such as temperament and maternal personality, may prove informative regarding their functional meaning and later consequences in terms of developmental outcomes.

Referential Emotion Processing and Social Learning

The studies reviewed above have tested infants' responses to isolated emotional facial expressions. However, in daily interactions emotional expressions very often refer to something or someone in the environment. Taking into account the referential nature of emotional facial expressions may help to determine the early precursors of social referencing and social learning. Furthermore, we may be able to assess infants' processing of the particular signal value of an emotional expression above and beyond pure perceptual discrimination.

Anger and fear are both emotional expressions of negative valence. However, their signal values and behavioral consequences for the observer are remarkably different and highly dependent on the referent of the emotional expression which may be signaled by the eye gaze direction of the face [Hoehl & Striano, 2008]. For instance, an angry face gazing straight ahead may signal immediate threat emanating from the emoter to the perceiver. A fearful face with gaze averted to the side may signal a common threat for the emoter and the perceiver in the environment. A fearful face gazing straight ahead, in contrast, may be rather ambiguous for the perceiver. In a series of experiments with adults, Adams and Kleck [2003] demonstrated that direct gaze speeds up recognition of faces expressing approach-related emotions (anger and happiness), whereas averted gaze speeds up recognition of avoidance-related emotional expressions (fear and sadness).

We used ERPs to test whether eye gaze direction affects how 7-month-old infants process angry and fearful facial expressions [Hoehl & Striano, 2008]. Infants saw angry and fearful faces with direct or averted gaze in a within-subjects design. Amplitude of the Nc component was significantly increased for angry faces gazing straight ahead compared to angry faces with averted gaze and fearful faces irrespective of gaze condition. This finding is consistent with an earlier report of increased brain responses for angry faces with direct versus averted gaze in 4-month-olds [Striano, Kopp, Grossmann & Reid, 2006]. It is also consistent with a greater Nc response for angry versus fearful faces with straight eye gaze previously found in the same age group [Kobiella, Grossmann, Reid & Striano, 2008]. Further support for infants' proposed sensitivity to the threat-related signal value of an angry face with straight gaze comes from a behavioral experiment with 5-month-olds. In this study, infants' eye blink startle reflex to loud noise was increased when viewing angry faces and reduced when viewing happy faces [Balaban, 1995]. In contrast to our results for angry faces, we found no significant effect of gaze direction on infants' brain responses to fearful faces. Thus, it seemed that 7-month-olds allocated increased attention to the most threatening stimuli in our experiment: angry faces gazing straight ahead.

We reasoned that a fearful face gazing to the side without a clear referent may still be highly ambiguous. We therefore conducted another experiment with fearful and neutral faces looking at small colorful objects presented directly next to the face [Hoehl, Palumbo, Heinisch & Striano, 2008]. As expected, infants responded with an increased Nc to fearful faces compared to neutral faces looking at an object at the side. A second group of infants saw the same neutral and fearful faces and peripheral objects; however, in this condition the faces were gazing straight ahead. No effect of emotion was found. A between-subjects comparison revealed that infants showed an increased Nc for fearful faces looking at a peripheral object compared to the same faces not cueing the object but gazing straight ahead. We concluded that 7-month-old infants are especially sensitive to fearful faces referring to something concrete in the environment [Hoehl, Palumbo, et al., 2008]. This fits well with results from a neuroimaging study with adults showing increased activity in the amygdala, a crucial structure for fear processing, in response to emotional faces directed at something in the environment compared to the faces alone [Hooker et al., 2006]. Although it is not clear to what extent the effect in 7-month-olds relies on deliberate rather than automatic processing of the emotional expression in combination with eye gaze, it is generally consistent with behavioral evidence for gradually developing joint attention skills between 7 and 10 months of age [Striano, Stahl & Cleveland, 2007], and infants' emerging social referencing behavior in ambiguous situations at the same age [Striano & Rochat, 2000; Striano & Vaish, 2006].

We later replicated this result with 6-month-olds [Hoehl & Striano, 2010a]. In this experiment, eyes were either directed at the object on one side of the face or towards empty space on the other side of the face. Again, we found an increased Nc amplitude for fearful faces looking at an object compared with fearful faces without a clear referent. This effect was not found in 3-month-olds, confirming that infants seem to become sensitive to fearful emotional expressions around 6 to 7 months of age [Peltola, Leppänen, Maki, et al., 2009]. In 9-month-olds we observed increased Nc amplitude for fearful versus neutral faces regardless of the referent of the expressions (i.e., regardless of whether the face looked towards the peripheral object or towards empty space). Thus, infants seem to become sensitive to fearful faces first when they refer to something in the environment around 6 months of age. Slightly later, at 9 months, infants' attention is increased for fearful versus neutral faces even when no immediate referent is present [Hoehl & Striano, 2010a]. Increased gaze following abilities emerging around the same age may contribute to this development. By 9–12 months of age, infants become less dependent on immediate referents of eye gaze cues and learn that eye gaze may be directed at more distant or not immediately visible targets [Butterworth, 1998; Moll & Tomasello, 2004].

The above-reviewed studies have shown that 6- and 7-month-old infants' processing of emotional expressions is affected by the eye gaze direction of the emoter and the presence or absence of referents of the expressions. The question arises whether infants' processing of novel objects is, in turn, affected by emotional expressions in combination with referential eye gaze cues. If a fearful face with eye gaze directed towards an object is a particularly salient stimulus, it could be expected that the object is subsequently more salient for the infant compared to an object that had been gaze cued with a neutral expression or not at all. Altered responses to objects associated with emotional expressions could be seen as an early indicator of social fear learning.

We tested this hypothesis in 3-, 6- and 9-month-old infants [Hoehl & Pauen, in preparation; Hoehl & Striano, 2010a; Hoehl, Wiese, et al., 2008]. Our initial hypothesis was that by the age of 6 months infants would show increased attention, as indicated by increased Nc amplitude, for objects that were gaze cued by a fearful face as compared to a neutral face. The same paradigm was used in all age groups: Infants saw a fearful or neutral face (within-subjects) looking at or looking away from (between-subjects) a colorful object that was displayed next to the face. Then, after a brief blank screen period, the object was presented again without the face and infants' ERP responses to the objects were measured. This paradigm allowed us to use the exact same object stimuli in all conditions. That is, ERPs were recorded to physically identical stimuli. Differences between conditions can only be explained in terms of the previous context: fearful or neutral face looking at (or looking away from) the object.

As expected, 6-month-olds showed an increased Nc response for objects that had been looked at by a face with a fearful versus neutral expression suggesting increased attention for potentially dangerous objects [Hoehl & Striano, 2010a]. No difference between objects in the fearful face condition versus the neutral face condition was found when faces looked away from the objects. That is, infants did not associate the expression with the object when the object was not referred to by the gaze direction of the face. In contrast to our initial hypothesis, however, we found the same effect in 3-month-old infants [Hoehl, Wiese, et al., 2008]. This is surprising, given that at 3 months of age infants do not show increased attention for fearful compared to happy or neutral faces. Possibly, very young infants already distinguish fearful faces from other expressions, but this is not displayed in their overt behavior or cortical responses. In adults, subcortical structures including the amygdala are involved in the processing of fearful faces [Vuilleumier, Armony, Driver & Dolan, 2003; Whalen et al., 1998]. Infants may respond to fearful faces on the subcortical level, invisible to EEG measurements of cortical activation. However, through the amygdala's connections to areas of the prefrontal cortex [Vuilleumier, 2005], this structure may affect the subsequent processing of fear-associated objects on the cortical level in very young infants.

Interestingly, surprised faces elicited the same effect as fearful faces in 3-month-olds [Hoehl & Pauen, 2011]. Similar to fearful faces, surprised faces are characterized by wide-opened eyes with a clearly visible sclera. Although fearful eyes alone do not elicit fear-like processing in 7-month-olds [Peltola, Leppänen, Vogel-Farley, et al., 2009], it may be very hard for 3-month-olds to distinguish between a fearful face and a surprised face because of their limited visual acuity [Salomao & Ventura, 1995]. Happy faces, in contrast, do not elicit increased attention towards objects in 3-month-olds, suggesting that the effect is not generalizable across all kinds of emotional expressions [Hoehl & Striano, 2010b].

Another surprising finding was that, in contrast to 6- and 3-month-olds, 9-month-olds did not show an increased Nc for objects cued by a fearful face [Hoehl & Striano, 2010a]. We speculated that 9-month-olds may already take into account the plausibility of an emotional expression in a given situation. Consequently, they did not respond to a fearful face looking at an obviously harmless colorful toy object, whereas younger infants may be more susceptible to others' emotional expressions. Around the age of 9 to 12 months infants reliably show overt social referencing in novel and ambiguous situations or when faced with a novel object [Campos, Thein & Owen,

2003; Striano & Rochat, 2000; Striano & Vaish, 2006]. That is, they turn to adults and adjust their own behavior according to the adult's emotional signals referring to the object or situation in question [Hertenstein & Campos, 2004; Moses, Baldwin, Rosicky & Tidball, 2001]. When the emotional expression is exaggerated or does not fit the situation (e.g., because the situation is unambiguous and not likely to elicit fear), infants have been reported to laugh or not respond to the emotional signals of adults [Campos et al., 2003]. It is not clear when in development infants start to be able to take into account the plausibility of an emotional reaction. It likely depends on how familiar the infant is with a given situation or kind of object.

In the last experiment of this series, we therefore used rather unfamiliar objects to test whether 9-month-olds would react with increased attention to them when the objects were cued by a fearful versus neutral face [Hoehl & Pauen, in preparation]. In this study, infants saw fearful and neutral faces looking towards spiders or perceptually matched flowers in a 2-by-2 within-subjects design. Spiders and flowers were then presented again and ERP responses were measured. Spiders are a rather unfamiliar stimulus category for infants (as opposed to flowers and, especially, toys) and may be associated with fear particularly easily because of an evolved preparedness [Mineka & Öhman, 2002]. We reasoned that a fearful face should affect 9-month-olds' responses to spiders more than their responses to less ambiguous flowers. As expected, we found an increased Nc for spiders that were cued by a fearful versus neutral face. As found for the toys in the previous study [Hoehl & Striano, 2010a], no effect of emotion condition was found for infants' responses to flowers.

In sum, it can be concluded that infants' processing of objects is affected by referential emotional expressions from very early on. Even 3-month-old infants direct increased attention towards a novel object that was just looked at by a fearful face [Hoehl, Wiese, et al., 2008]. In 3-month-olds, however, this response seems to be rather unspecific. Infants at this age show the same effect for surprised faces looking at objects [Hoehl & Pauen, 2011]. In 9-month-olds, in contrast, this effect is very specific. Nine-month-olds do not show the effect when unambiguous toys or flowers are used as stimuli [Hoehl & Pauen, in preparation; Hoehl & Striano, 2010a], and they do not show an effect when surprised faces are presented [Hoehl & Pauen, 2011]. They do, however, direct increased attention to pictures of spiders that were just looked at by a fearful versus neutral face [Hoehl & Pauen, in preparation], suggesting that their attention towards objects is particularly affected by fearful facial expressions when the referents of the emotion are ambiguous and/or potentially threatening and fear-relevant.

Infants' Scanning Patterns of Emotional Faces as Assessed by Eye Tracking

Recently, researchers have started to use eye tracking to examine infants' scanning patterns for different facial emotional expressions. As opposed to more conventional manual coding of infants' looking behavior based on video recordings, modern remote eye tracking systems allow for very precise measurements of infants' visual scanning patterns.

Hunnius and colleagues measured 4- and 7-month-olds' and adults' scanning patterns when viewing five different emotional expressions: angry, fearful, happy, sad, and neutral [Hunnius et al., 2011]. All age groups showed differential scanning of threat-related (i.e., fearful and angry) versus non-threat-related expressions (i.e., happy, sad, neutral), which was characterized by less fixating on and less scanning of the inner features of the face. This was termed a 'vigilant' or avoidant style of looking at faces with angry and fearful expressions. In addition, adults, but not infants avoided eye contact with angry and fearful faces. Overall, adults showed more focused scanning of emotional faces than infants by fixating on the inner features including eyes and mouths. In contrast, infants' fixations were more scattered across the stimuli, and they rarely fixated on the mouth region. The authors conclude that avoidant looking patterns to threat-related expressions seem to emerge early in life, whereas eye contact avoidance seems to be a learned response only to be found later in development.

Another study using eye tracking was conducted by Peltola, Leppänen, Vogel-Farley, et al. [2009]. They showed 7-month-old infants happy, neutral, and fearful faces, as well as neutral faces with fearful eyes. In contrast to Hunnius et al. [2011], the authors report no differences in scanning patterns by specific emotional expression. Similar to the results reported by Hunnius et al. [2011], however, infants spent the most time scanning the eye region when compared to the other areas of the face including the mouth.

We recently used eye tracking to examine 7-month-olds' visual scanning of five emotional expressions (angry, fearful, happy, neutral, sad) depending on the gaze direction of the face (direct gaze versus averted gaze) [Hoehl & Koch, unpubl. data]. One male and one female actor displayed each emotional expression and gaze direction. Thirty-one infants (average age 7 months, 14 days; 11 females) took part in this experiment using a Tobii T 60 eye tracker. Relative fixation length was taken as dependent measure and 5 areas of interest (AOIs) were chosen which were equally large for each emotion and gaze condition: whole face, inner features (covering eyes, nose and mouth), eyes, nose, and mouth. Similar to Peltola et al. [2009], we found no differences in fixation length across conditions when looking at the complete face, all $p > 0.30$. Furthermore, when testing for differences between infants' fixations across three nonoverlapping AOIs covering eyes, nose, and mouth, respectively, infants explored the eye region the longest, $F_{(2,29)} = 29$, $p < 0.001$. There was also a significant interaction between AOI and emotion, $F_{(8,23)} = 5.8$, $p < 0.001$.

Infants fixated on the eye region significantly less for fearful faces than for all the other emotional expressions, $F_{(4,27)} = 7.90$, $p < 0.001$ (pairwise two-tailed comparisons between fearful eyes vs. all other emotions, all $p < 0.01$, Bonferroni corrections were applied). This was found regardless of eye gaze direction as no main effect or interaction involving this factor was observed. Together with the findings by Peltola, Leppänen, Vogel-Farley, et al. [2009], our results suggest that the eye region is not the critical feature for infants' identification of fearful faces.

The mouth region, in contrast, was fixated on significantly longer when fearful and angry faces were shown compared with happy and sad faces, $F_{(4,27)} = 6.90$, $p = 0.001$ (pairwise two-tailed comparisons between fearful and angry mouths vs. happy and sad mouths, all $p < 0.03$, Bonferroni corrections were applied). Thus, although our results require replication, infants may depend on the mouth region more than on the eye region when processing threat-related facial expressions.

Finally, we looked at differences across emotional expressions and gaze directions for an AOI covering the inner features of the faces (including eyes, nose, and mouth). A main effect was found for emotion condition, $F_{(4,27)} = 3.20$, $p = 0.03$. This effect was due to shorter fixation lengths for happy faces compared to fearful and neutral faces (pairwise two-tailed comparisons, all $p < 0.03$, Bonferroni corrections were applied). The latter finding is consistent with the typically reported visual preference for fearful over happy faces in 7-month-olds (see discussion above). We did not, however, replicate the avoidant or vigilant scanning pattern for threat-related expressions observed by Hunnius et al. [2011].

Given that the few studies conducted so far have yielded inconsistent results, more research on infants' visual scanning of emotional facial expressions is needed using eye tracking. In particular, dynamic expressions and emotional expressions in complex environments including specific referents may be used to get a clearer and more ecologically valid picture of young infants' looking behavior and decoding of emotional faces. This research should also be expanded to younger and older infants to be able to gain a developmental perspective. It will be especially interesting to test infants between 5 and 7 months – the age when attention biases to fearful over happy and neutral faces typically emerge [Peltola, Leppänen, Maki, et al., 2009]. Changes in looking patterns during this age range may help reveal the mechanisms underlying this development.

Conclusions and Future Directions

In the present chapter, I have reviewed classic and modern approaches to studying infants' processing of emotional facial expressions. Whereas classic paradigms have allowed for testing infants' abilities to discriminate and categorize emotional expressions, novel approaches have enabled us to go beyond purely perceptual discrimination to get clues about infants' processing of the signal values of different expressions. For instance, direct eye gaze increases 7-month-olds' attention to angry faces [Hoehl & Striano, 2008], whereas attention towards fearful faces is increased when eye gaze is directed at a referent in the environment in infants of the same age [Hoehl, Palumbo, et al., 2008], suggesting that infants process eye gaze in combination with emotional facial expression to quickly detect threat.

A range of studies conducted at different laboratories has demonstrated that infants' attention bias for fearful faces over happy faces seems to emerge by 7 months of age [de Haan et al., 2004; Kotsoni et al., 2001; Ludemann & Nelson, 1988; Nelson & Dolgin, 1985; Peltola, Leppänen, Maki, et al., 2009]. The mechanisms of the development of this bias and its function will be subject to further investigation. For instance, cross-cultural work is clearly warranted to test the supposed association of this bias with infants' ability to locomote and prior experiences with emotional expressions. Infants may be tested in cultures in which gross motor abilities on average develop earlier or later than in Western societies.

Furthermore, studies have related individual differences in emotional face processing to genetic polymorphisms, infant temperament, and maternal personality [de Haan et al., 2004; Grossmann et al., 2011; Leppänen et al., 2011]. Longitudinal research will provide crucial information on the functional relevance of infants' early attention biases and their implications for developmental outcomes such as emotion regulation abilities. For instance, some infants' difficulties in disengaging from a negative stimulus [Leppänen et al., 2011] may predict their later vulnerability for affective disorders, especially depression, which has been linked to a negativity bias in directing attention to emotional stimuli [Browning, Holmes & Harmer, 2010].

Finally, eye tracking and neurophysiological measures will be increasingly used to trace the early origins of infants' emotional learning and social referencing. Initial studies suggest that infants take into account the referential nature of emotional facial expressions and eye gaze cues very early in development. Emotional expressions affect object processing as early as 3 months after birth [Hoehl, Wiese, et al., 2008]. By 9 months of age, infants seem to associate fear rather specifically with unfamiliar and potentially threatening objects [Hoehl & Pauen, in preparation]. The combined use of more than one technology in the same study (e.g., eye tracking and EEG) will likely advance our understanding of infant emotion processing. For instance, fine-grained analyses of infants' looking patterns may provide information on their referential eye gaze processing in relation to an object and predict neurophysiological responses to the object. Further research, for instance, using head-mounted eye-tracking [Franchak, Kretch, Soska & Adolph, 2011] and gaze-contingent paradigms [Deligianni, Senju, Gergely & Csibra, 2011], will help to determine infants' scanning patterns and information gathering in complex and ecologically valid social learning situations.

References

Adams, R.B., Jr., & Kleck, R.E. (2003). Perceived gaze direction and the processing of facial displays of emotion. *Psychological Science, 14*, 644–647.

Balaban, M.T. (1995). Affective influences on startle in five-month-old infants: Reactions to facial expressions of emotions. *Child Develelopment, 66*, 28–36.

Barrera, M.E., & Maurer, D. (1981). The perception of facial expressions by the three-month-old. *Child Develelopment, 52*, 203–206.

Browning, M., Holmes, E.A., & Harmer, C.J. (2010). The modification of attentional bias to emotional information: A review of the techniques, mechanisms, and relevance to emotional disorders. *Cogn Affect Behav Neurosci, 10*, 8–20.

Butterworth, G. (1998). Origins of joint visual attention in infancy. *Monogr Soc Res Child Dev, 63*, 144–166.

Campos, J.J., Anderson, David I., Barbu-Roth, Marianne A., Hubbard, Edward M., Hertenstein, Matthew J., & Witherington, David. (2000). Travel Broadens the Mind. *Infancy, 1*, 149–219.

Campos, J.J., Thein, S., & Owen, D. (2003). A Darwinian legacy to understanding human infancy – Emotional expressions as behavior regulators. *Annals of the New York Academy of Sciences, 1000*, 110–134.

Cicchetti, D., & Curtis, W.J. (2005). An event-related potential study of the processing of affective facial expressions in young children who experienced maltreatment during the first year of life. *Developmental Psychopathology, 17*, 641–677.

de Haan, M., Belsky, J., Reid, V., Volein, A., & Johnson, M.H. (2004). Maternal personality and infants' neural and visual responsivity to facial expressions of emotion. *Journal of Child Psychology and Psychiatry, 45*, 1209–1218.

de Haan, M., & Nelson, C.A. (1998). Discrimination and categorisation of facial expressions of emotion during infancy. In A. Slater (Ed.), *Perceptual development.* Hove, UK: Psychology Press.

Deligianni, F., Senju, A., Gergely, G., & Csibra, G. (2011). Automated gaze-contingent objects elicit orientation following in 8-month-old infants. *Developmental Psychology, 47*, 1499–1503.

Farroni, Teresa, Menon, Enrica, Rigato, Silvia, & Johnson, Mark H. (2007). The perception of facial expressions in newborns. *European Journal of Developmental Psychology, 4*, 2–13.

Franchak, J.M., Kretch, K.S., Soska, K.C., & Adolph, K.E. (2011). Head-mounted eye tracking: A new method to describe infant looking. *Child Develelopment, 82*, 1738–1750.

Grossmann, T., Johnson, M.H., Vaish, A., Hughes, D.A., Quinque, D., Stoneking, M., & Friederici, A.D. (2011). Genetic and neural dissociation of individual responses to emotional expressions in human infants. *Developmental Cognitive Neuroscience, 1*, 57–66.

Grossmann, T., Striano, T., & Friederici, A.D. (2007). Developmental changes in infants' processing of happy and angry facial expressions: A neurobehavioral study. *Brain and Cognition, 64*, 30–41.

Hertenstein, M.J., & Campos, J.J. (2004). The retention effects of an adult's emotional displays on infant behavior. *Child Development, 75*, 595–613.

Hoehl, S. (2008). The perception of emotional expressions in infancy. In T. Striano & V.M. Reid (Eds.), *Social Cognition: Development, Neuroscience, and Autism.* Oxford: Social Cognition: Development, Neuroscience, and Autism.

Hoehl, S., Palumbo, L., Heinisch, C., & Striano, T. (2008). Infants' attention is biased by emotional expressions and eye gaze direction. *Neuroreport, 19*, 579–582.

Hoehl, S., & Pauen, S. (2011). Do surprised faces affect infants' attention toward novel objects? *Neuroreport, 22*, 906–910.

Hoehl, S., & Pauen, S. (in preparation). Infants' preparedness to identify fear-inducing stimuli.

Hoehl, S., Reid, V., Mooney, J., & Striano, T. (2008). What are you looking at? Infants' neural processing of an adult's object-directed eye gaze. *Developmental Science, 11*, 10–16.

Hoehl, S., & Striano, T. (2008). Neural processing of eye gaze and threat-related emotional facial expressions in infancy. *Child Development, 79*, 1752–1760.

Hoehl, S., & Striano, T. (2010a). The development of emotional face and eye gaze processing. *Developmental Science, 13*, 813–825.

Hoehl, S., & Striano, T. (2010b). Infants' neural processing of positive emotion and eye gaze. *Social Neuroscience, 5*, 30–39.

Hoehl, S., Wiese, L., & Striano, T. (2008). Young infants' neural processing of objects is affected by eye gaze direction and emotional expression. *PLoS One, 3*, e2389.

Hooker, C.I., Germine, L.T., Knight, R.T., & D'Esposito, M. (2006). Amygdala response to facial expressions reflects emotional learning. *Journal of Neuroscience, 26*, 8915–8922.

Hunnius, S., de Wit, T.C., Vrins, S., & von Hofsten, C. (2011). Facing threat: Infants' and adults' visual scanning of faces with neutral, happy, sad, angry, and fearful emotional expressions. *Cognition and Emotion, 25*, 193–205.

Kobiella, Andrea, Grossmann, Tobias, Reid, Vincent M., & Striano, T. (2008). The discrimination of angry and fearful facial expressions in 7-month-old infants: An event-related potential study. *Cognition and Emotion, 22*, 134–146.

Kotsoni, E., de Haan, M., & Johnson, M.H. (2001). Categorical perception of facial expressions by 7-month-old infants. *Perception, 30*, 1115–1125.

LaBarbera, J.D., Izard, C.E., Vietze, P., & Parisi, S.A. (1976). Four- and six-month-old infants' visual responses to joy, anger, and neutral expressions. *Child Develelopment, 47*, 535–538.

Leppänen, J.M., & Nelson, C.A. (2006). The development and neural bases of facial emotion recognition. *Advances in Child Development and Behavior, 34*, 207–246.

Leppänen, J.M., & Nelson, C.A. (2009). Tuning the developing brain to social signals of emotions. *Nature Reviews Neuroscience, 10*, 37–47.

Leppänen, J.M., Peltola, M.J., Puura, K., Mantymaa, M., Mononen, N., & Lehtimaki, T. (2011). Serotonin and early cognitive development: Variation in the tryptophan hydroxylase 2 gene is associated with visual attention in 7-month-old infants. *Journal of Child Psychology and Psychiatry, 52*, 1144–1152.

Ludemann, P., & Nelson, C.A. (1988). Categorical representation of facial expressions by 7-month-old infants. *Developmental Psychology, 24*, 492–501.

Mineka, S., & Öhman, A. (2002). Phobias and preparedness: The selective, automatic, and encapsulated nature of fear. *Biological Psychiatry, 52,* 927–937.

Moll, H., & Tomasello, M. (2004). 12- and 18-month-old infants follow gaze to spaces behind barriers. *Developmental Science, 7,* F1–F9.

Moses, L.J., Baldwin, D.A., Rosicky, J.G., & Tidball, G. (2001). Evidence for referential understanding in the emotions domain at twelve and eighteen months. *Child Development, 72,* 718–735.

Nelson, C.A., & de Haan, M. (1996). Neural correlates of infants' visual responsiveness to facial expressions of emotion. *Developmental Psychobiology, 29,* 577–595.

Nelson, C.A., & Dolgin, K.G. (1985). The generalized discrimination of facial expressions by seven-month-old infants. *Child Development, 56,* 58–61.

Parker, S.W., & Nelson, C.A. (2005). The impact of early institutional rearing on the ability to discriminate facial expressions of emotion: An event-related potential study. *Child Development, 76,* 54–72.

Peltola, M.J., Leppänen, J.M., Maki, S., & Hietanen, J.K. (2009). Emergence of enhanced attention to fearful faces between 5 and 7 months of age. *Social Cognitive and Affective Neuroscience, 4,* 134–142.

Peltola, M.J., Leppänen, J.M., Palokangas, T., & Hietanen, J.K. (2008). Fearful faces modulate looking duration and attention disengagement in 7-month-old infants. *Developmental Science, 11,* 60–68.

Peltola, M.J., Leppänen, J.M., Vogel-Farley, V.K., Hietanen, J.K., & Nelson, C.A. (2009). Fearful faces but not fearful eyes alone delay attention disengagement in 7-month-old infants. *Emotion, 9,* 560–565.

Pollak, S.D., Cicchetti, D., Hornung, K., & Reed, A. (2000). Recognizing emotion in faces: developmental effects of child abuse and neglect. *Developmental Psychology, 36,* 679–688.

Pollak, S.D., Klorman, R., Thatcher, J.E., & Cicchetti, D. (2001). P3b reflects maltreated children's reactions to facial displays of emotion. *Psychophysiology, 38,* 267–274.

Reynolds, G.D., & Richards, J.E. (2005). Familiarization, attention, and recognition memory in infancy: An event-related potential and cortical source localization study. *Developmental Psychology, 41,* 598–615.

Richards, J.E. (2003). Attention affects the recognition of briefly presented visual stimuli in infants: an ERP study. *Developmental Science, 6,* 312–328.

Salomao, S.R., & Ventura, D.F. (1995). Large sample population age norms for visual acuities obtained with Vistech-Teller Acuity Cards. *Investigative Ophthalmology & Visual Science, 36,* 657–670.

Striano, T., Kopp, F., Grossmann, T., & Reid, V.M. (2006). Eye contact influences neural processing of emotional expressions in 4-month-old infants. *Social Cognitive & Affective Neuroscience, 1,* 87–94.

Striano, T., & Rochat, P. (2000). Emergence of selective social referencing in infancy. *Infancy, 1,* 253–264.

Striano, T., Stahl, D., & Cleveland, A. (2007). Taking a closer look at social and cognitive skills: A weekly longitudinal assessment between 7 and 10 months of age. *European Journal of Developmental Psychology, 6,* 567–591.

Striano, T., & Vaish, A. (2006). Seven- to 9-month-old infants use facial expressions to interpret others' actions. *British Journal of Developmental Psychology, 24,* 753–760.

Vaish, A., Grossmann, T., & Woodward, A. (2008). Not all emotions are created equal: The negativity bias in social-emotional development. *Psychological Bulletin, 134,* 383–403.

Vuilleumier, P. (2005). How brains beware: neural mechanisms of emotional attention. *Trends in Cognitive Sciences, 9,* 585–594.

Vuilleumier, P., Armony, J.L., Driver, J., & Dolan, R.J. (2003). Distinct spatial frequency sensitivities for processing faces and emotional expressions. *Nature Neuroscience, 6,* 624–631.

Walker-Andrews, A.S. (1997). Infants' perception of expressive behaviors: Differentiation of multimodal information. *Psychological Bulletin, 121,* 437–456.

Whalen, P.J., Rauch, S.L., Etcoff, N.L., McInerney, S.C., Lee, M.B., & Jenike, M.A. (1998). Masked presentations of emotional facial expressions modulate amygdala activity without explicit knowledge. *Journal of Neuroscience, 18,* 411–418.

Wilcox, B.M., & Clayton, F.L. (1968). Infant visual fixation on motion pictures of the human face. *Journal of Experimental Child Psychology, 6,* 22–32.

Young-Browne, G., Rosenfeld, H.M., & Horowitz, F.D. (1977). Infant discrimination of facial expressions. *Child Development, 48,* 555–562.

Stefanie Hoehl
Institute of Psychology, Heidelberg University
Hauptstrasse 47/51
DE-69117 Heidelberg (Germany)
E-Mail stefanie.hoehl@psychologie.uni-heidelberg.de

Hansen Lagattuta K (ed): Children and Emotion. New Insights into Developmental Affective Sciences.
Contrib Hum Dev. Basel, Karger, 2014, vol 26, pp 13–28 (DOI: 10.1159/000354347)

Developmental Affective Psychophysiology: Using Physiology to Inform Our Understanding of Emotional Development

Paul D. Hastings · Sarah S. Kahle · Georges H.-P. Han
University of California, Davis, Calif., USA

Abstract

There has been a marked shift in the study of emotional development in recent years, as increasing numbers of laboratories and researchers have incorporated assessments of biological activity into their efforts to understand emotional development. In this chapter, we briefly describe several established and emergent psychophysiological techniques, with examples of how researchers have used neurophysiological, neuroendocrinological, autonomic, and electromyographic measures to provide new insights into children's emotions. We identify a number of issues and questions that have long posed challenges to the psychophysiological study of emotional development, and highlight our own recent and ongoing efforts to address these challenges in our studies of emotion regulation, expression and experience.

In the past two decades, a surge of exciting and innovative psychophysiological research has enlivened the study of emotional development. With the advent of new technologies, new theories, new journals, and renewed appreciation from developmental scientists for the importance of both emotional and neurobiological processes, developmental affective psychophysiology has emerged as a dynamic field of work [e.g., Barrett, Fox, Morgan, Fidler & Daunhauer, 2013; Dennis, Buss & Hastings, 2012].

We begin with a brief overview of neurobiological techniques and technologies being used by developmental scientists to study emotion. This is followed by consideration of several perpetually vexing conundrums in the application of psychophysiology to the study of children's emotional development. We then review some of our efforts to address these issues and highlight some potentially informative future directions for research. Throughout, our goal is to capture readers' excitement about the new possibilities that are unearthed by research that is conducted at the interfaces of psychophysiological, affective, and developmental processes.

And by *Emotion*, We Mean…

As most emotion researchers seem compelled to do, we first provide the definitions of *emotion* and associated constructs that guide our work. From functional and evolutionary theories of emotion, there is growing consensus that emotions are biologically-prepared adaptive processes [Cole, Martin & Dennis, 2004; Dennis et al., 2012]. Emotions of varying valence and intensity are experienced in rapid response to stimuli or situations, contributing to the meaning or relevance assigned to those triggers. Emotions prime action patterns or behavioral response tendencies for dealing effectively with these cues and the contexts within which they are experienced [Bradley & Lang, 2007], sustaining favorable conditions that support well-being or changing unfavorable conditions that undermine it. Thus, emotions are integrative multi-faceted processes, drawing on neurobiological, perceptual, cognitive, and behavioral systems that serve individuals' contextually bound goals [Thompson, 2011a].

From this perspective, emotions regulate cognition and behavior. Yet, emotions themselves also get regulated. Careful consideration has been given to how (or even, whether) *emotions* can be distinguished from, and understood in relation to, *emotion regulation* [Cole et al., 2004; Thompson, 2011b]. Emotion regulation encompasses both automatic and deliberate processes, from both internal sources and external agents that modify the dynamic aspects of how emotions are experienced and expressed. Emotion regulation can involve the delay or acceleration, muting or exaggeration, and termination or maintenance of the arousal, feelings, thoughts, and actions that comprise an elicited emotion.

Effective emotion regulation enhances the degree to which an emotion facilitates one's attainment of goals in the eliciting context. This can promote well-being and adaptive engagement with the social environment, but the immediate or enduring outcomes of discrete emotion regulation events are not always beneficial. One's goals might not be concordant with others' expectations for appropriate or acceptable actions, as with, for example, a goal of magnifying an angry display in order to intimidate a peer and obtain a desired toy. Similarly, one might regulate emotion to adapt to a context that is atypical of venues supporting well-being, say, monitoring for anger cues in a home with a violent caregiver [Strang, Hanson & Pollak, 2012]. Thus, a child's immediate efforts to regulate emotion might be seen as *dys*regulated by others, and even if such efforts are 'functional' for attaining a short-term goal, they might also convey undesirable consequences in the future.

The temporal dimension also underlies variation in how the term emotion regulation is used. Regulating a discrete emotional *state* can be distinguished from emotion regulation as a *trait*, or the tendency to be more or less emotionally well-regulated, across time and situations [Rutter & Sroufe, 2000]. Thus, one can be regulating well, in the moment, or be an emotionally well-regulated individual, in general. Similarly, short-lived, or phasic, emotional states are distinct from more enduring, or tonic, affective conditions and characteristics. Moods are emotional conditions that can persist for more extended periods, from several minutes to several days. Paralleling trait emotion regulation, emotional aspects of temperament reflect the early-developing and moderately stable tendencies of individuals to respond to stimuli and situations more positively or more negatively, and with greater or lesser intensity [Shiner et al., 2012]. Finally, the study of development, emotion and neurobiology can be extended to chronic emotional difficulties and disorders, such as depression, anxiety problems, and the emotional aspects of disruptive behavior disorders. Together, emotions, emotion regulation, moods, temperament and emotional problems constitute the affective targets of study that are examined in developmental affective psychophysiology.

Targets of Technology: Measurements from Heads, Hormones, Hearts, and Hands

Developmental scientists interested in emotion have targeted several neurobiological systems, reflecting the multiple levels of physiological activity involved in emotional processes. The brain communicates with the rest of the body to prepare one for responding to salient cues, to convey emotional arousal through expressions, or to prime other motor action patterns. Studying hormone levels and somatic activity produced by peripheral nervous systems is integral to understanding emotional development.

Neurophysiology

Given that emotions involve attention towards, assessment of, and response to personally salient stimuli, it follows that meta-analytic reviews of neuroimaging studies of emotion have shown that neural activity associated with emotion is widely distributed throughout the brain [Murphy, Nimmo-Smith & Lawrence, 2003]. However, certain regions have been consistently identified and appear to be most central to affective processes [Bradley & Lang, 2007; Vytal & Hamaan, 2010]. That is, there is overwhelming evidence that the amygdala and surrounding limbic system play primary roles in fear arousal, as well as other emotions; numerous regions within the prefrontal cortex have been implicated in emotion regulation, and the striatum appears critical for linking emotional cues with behavioral responses of approaching versus avoiding. It is increasingly evident that rather than studying neural activity as isolated within distinct brain regions, researchers must examine the systemic coordination of activity across brain regions to understand the complexity of emotional neurophysiology; numerous neural networks of emotion have been identified or proposed [e.g., Dennis, O'Toole & DiCicco, 2013].

Affective neurophysiology has predominantly been studied in adults, and the key systems and processes may differ in infants, children, and adolescents. Neural development continues throughout at least the first quarter century of life, with the pace of maturation varying across neural regions [Giedd & Rapoport, 2010]. For example, striatal and limbic regions involved in reward processing and appetitive motivation mature rapidly in early and mid-adolescence, whereas prefrontal regions involved in regulating these drives have a slower course of maturation that extends into adulthood. These divergent trajectories are thought to contribute to heightened emotionality and impulsivity in adolescence [Casey, Getz & Galvan, 2008]. Similarly, across age groups, there are distinctions and overlaps in the neural regions involved in recognizing others' distress [Decety & Michalska, 2010], which could reflect developmental changes in the regulation of empathic arousal [Hastings, Miller, Kahle & Zahn-Waxler, 2014]. The paucity of longitudinal research on affective neurophysiology, however, limits our ability to infer how developments in brain structure and activity correspond with changes in emotion experience and regulation.

Numerous techniques for studying emotional neurophysiology are appropriate for developmental research [see also Hoehl, this vol.; Perez-Edgar et al., this vol.]. Electroencephalography (EEG) and event-related potentials (ERP) assess cortical neural activity and offer excellent temporal information on brain activity, but limited spatial resolution. Several EEG studies have shown that children with fearful or inhibited temperaments show asymmetrical EEG activity: relatively greater activity in the right than left frontal hemispheres likely reflects a neural bias toward negative emotionality and greater motivation to withdraw than approach [Miskovic & Schmidt, 2012]. Recent ERP research linked inhibited temperament with state emotion regulation; examining the late positive potential showed that more fearful young children were less able to implement the top-down regulatory strategy of emotional reappraisal to decrease their attention to unpleasant stimuli [DeCicco, Solomon & Dennis, 2012].

Structural and functional magnetic resonance imaging (MRI) has been increasingly used with children, providing greater spatial clarity albeit more limited temporal resolution than EEG or ERP. The size, noise, and restrictions on movement imposed by MRI machines can be intimidating for children, but careful methodological efforts can establish children's comfort. Additional neuroimaging technologies, including near-infrared spectroscopy and diffusion tensor imaging (DTI), also advance the tool-kit that researchers have for studying how the developing brain is involved in emotional development. Near-infrared spectroscopy offers lower spatial resolution of gray matter than MRI, but the equipment is portable and less intimidating, such that it can be implemented in a wider variety of venues. DTI creates images of white matter, which supports neural communication and has a prolonged maturational course of development and distribution. Functional MRI research has shown stronger connectivity between the ACC and amygdala in adults than in children in response to anger provocations, suggesting a long maturational course for prefrontal contributions to emotion regulation [Perlman & Pelphrey, 2011]. Similarly, a DTI study also provided evidence that white matter supported connectivity between prefrontal cortex regions that was in turn linked to effective self-regulatory behavior in children [Madsen et al., 2010].

The evidence for convergent findings across neuroimaging techniques is promising, and one of the exciting new ventures in developmental neuroscience involves combining complimentary procedures to glean greater understanding of dynamic emotional processes within the brain. Applying integrative and innovative approaches to projects with developmentally informed designs will advance our ability to study the multiple levels and kinds of brain structure and activity that contribute to emotions in children and youth.

Neuroendocrinology

Hormones are chemical messengers secreted into the circulatory system that can take several seconds to several minutes to reach their target tissues and produce effects. The hypothalamic-pituitary-adrenal (HPA) axis is the neuroendocrine system most commonly studied by developmental scientists. The HPA axis has many metabolic and regulatory functions, including regulation of stress responses [Gunnar & Adam, 2012; Kaltas & Chrousos, 2007]. Perceptions of physical and psychological threats to the self can induce acute HPA responses, which ultimately result in cortisol and dehydroepiandrosterone being secreted into the serum of the circulatory system, where they are carried by the blood to targets throughout the body to produce a variety of effects. In addition to being acutely responsive to discrete events or salient cues, the HPA axis follows a circadian cycle of activity, from an early morning peak (cortisol awakening response, CAR) to a zenith in the evening. This circadian rhythm constitutes 'baseline' or 'basal' HPA activity.

Stress reactivity and regulation are not synonymous with emotion reactivity and regulation, and not all emotional stimuli trigger HPA responses [Gunnar & Adam, 2012]. Emotions that reflect negative self-evaluation or feeling threatened, such as shame, loneliness, anxiety and fear, are most reliably associated with acute elevations in salivary cortisol, across ages. For example, preschoolers had larger and more prolonged cortisol elevations when they showed more shame after failing to accomplish a supposedly easy task; cortisol was not related to displays of sadness [Mills, Imm, Walling & Weiler, 2008]. Examining time scales in emotional processes, Adam [2012] collected multiple saliva samples and self-reports of loneliness from adolescents over several days. More loneliness one day predicted stronger CAR the next. The CAR is thought to provide an 'energy boost' to engage with the social world, such that stronger CAR may reflect physiological regulation to combat lonely moods. This work, however, also revealed the double-edged sword of acute emotion regulation alluded to earlier. Over the subsequent year, youths with larger CAR were more likely to experience major depressive disorder – independent of their earlier loneliness or depression symptoms. Perhaps repeated expenditures of resources to overcome loneliness took their toll on these youths, as chronically elevated cortisol levels can have neurotoxic effects [Kaltas & Chrousos, 2007].

The HPA axis and cortisol are not the only hormonal targets of interest for emotion researchers. There also has been considerable study of sex hormones, such as testosterone and estradiol, produced by the hypothalamic-pituitary-gonadal axis, and neuropeptides, like oxytocin and vasopressin which are important regulators of social affiliation. For example, intranasal administration of oxytocin to fathers of infants has been found to increase fathers' autonomic regulation (higher respiratory sinus arrhythmia, RSA; see below) and positive engagement with infants during play, and infants' RSA and social engagement behaviors increased in parallel [Feldman, 2012a].

Autonomic Physiology

Modulations in somatic arousal help prepare the body to act, including regulating the experience of emotions, and communicating emotional states to social partners. The autonomic nervous system (ANS) rapidly and bidirectionally conveys emotional information between the brain and the body. Neural activity associated with perception of, attention to, and processing of affective stimuli triggers ANS activity. Feedback from peripheral systems modulates neural activity and affects emotional experience, expression, and regulation [Critchley, 2005; Porges, 2007]. Effective and continual communication between central and peripheral systems is an essential element of emotion.

The sympathetic (SNS) and parasympathetic (PNS) branches of the ANS coordinate autonomic changes [Berntson, Quigley & Lozano, 2007], and different peripheral measures offer varying degrees of confidence for determining which branch is responsible for measured activity. Determining whether autonomic changes are driven by sympathetic or parasympathetic control is important for understanding emotional physiology. SNS and PNS stimulation tend to have opposite effects on autonomic arousal, with greater SNS activation accompanying increased autonomic arousal and greater PNS activation accompanying decreased autonomic arousal. This classical homeostatic or antagonistic model offers too simplistic a portrayal of the ANS, though, as the PNS and SNS can be reciprocally, independently, or jointly active. The terms *autonomic space* and *allodynamic control* are used to characterize the simultaneous and joint contributions of SNS and PNS stimulation to somatic activity [Berntson & Cacioppo, 2007]. As we face the changing demands of what is encountered in our daily activities, adaptive functioning is maintained by continually adjusting the activity levels of our physiological states (allostasis).

The SNS is part of the body's rapid stress-response system, the sympathetic adrenomedullary system. In addition to directly enervating several tissues, the SNS stimulates the adrenal medulla to release norepinephrine and epinephrine, which drive the fight-or-flight responses of many tissues. The SNS has been closely linked to the arousal of both anger and fear, as well as emotionally motivated behavioral response patterns of activation/approach and inhibition/withdrawal [Fowles, 1988]. SNS activity can be measured through several indices, including cardiac pre-ejection period (PEP), skin conductance levels or electrodermal response, and salivary levels of the enzyme alpha-amylase. Using the Trier Social Stress Test to evoke anxiety, de Veld, Riksen-Walraven and de Weerth [2012] showed that reduced salivary alpha-amylase reactivity, and faster recovery were linked with children's reported use of more suppression to control their emotions, but not their use of re-appraisal. Suppression has been considered a less mature or adaptive emotion regulation strategy than reappraisal [Gullone, Hughes, King & Tonge, 2010], but it is possible that children find suppression to be more effective for controlling arousal when coping with an inescapable anxiety-inducing situation.

Developmental and emotional study of the PNS has mainly focused on quantifying the chronotropic influence of the vagus nerve, or 10th cranial nerve, on heart rate. The component of heart rate variability called RSA, or cardiac vagal tone, is a useful marker of individual differences in the ability to regulate emotional arousal [Beauchaine, 2001]. Porges' polyvagal theory [2007] holds that higher basal RSA supports a greater capacity to exert parasympathetic control over autonomic activity, increasing or decreasing arousal in order to cope with emotional challenges. In safe situations, higher RSA (applying the 'vagal brake' on arousal) helps one to calmly engage in positive social interactions. When an important event occurs, modest withdrawal of PNS influence, indexed by decreasing RSA (releasing the 'brake'), increases orientation and attention. Stronger withdrawal of PNS influence in response to an event suggests a potential threat or challenge requiring a larger increase in arousal (the fight-or-flight response). An important tenet of polyvagal theory is that effective parasympathetic regulation necessitates flexibly suppressing or augmenting RSA in accord with contextual cues [Beauchaine, 2012]. For example, Calkins and colleagues found that preschoolers demonstrated higher performance on tests of executive function if they had modest RSA suppression (orienting) than if they had either stronger suppression (threatened) or augmentation (failure to focus) [Marcovitch et al., 2010]. In contrast, during a frustrating impossible puzzle task, preschoolers who showed less RSA suppression (or more augmentation) more often self-regulated by re-directing attention [Perry, Calkins, Nelson, Leerkes & Marcovitch, 2012]. Stronger RSA suppression might have supported a more sustained, but fruitless, engagement with the frustrating activity.

Skeletomotor Physiology

The skeletomotor system is implicated in muscular control and, with the ANS, is critical for neural responses to emotional cues being transformed into adaptive motor response patterns [Tassinary, Cacioppo & Vanman, 2007]. Psychophysiological researchers have used electromyography to record minute movements of muscles through adhesive electrodes on the skin, which are produced during cognitive and affective activity even without conscious awareness. Dozens of muscles are involved in facial expressions of emotions, and measuring movements that are not visually perceptible can reveal when stimuli have evoked an affective response that might otherwise go unrecognized. For example, in research with infants, children, and adolescents, the eye-blink startle response, which varies across temperaments and is linked to amygdala activity, shows sensitivity to the emotional valence of visual stimuli [Fox, Kirwan & Reeb-Sutherland, 2012]. Schmitz et al. [2011] found that 7- to 17-year-old girls showed a greater potentiation of eye-blink startle to negatively valenced stimuli presented on a random, unpredictable schedule than did boys, which could reflect an early-emerging gender difference in susceptibility to elevated anxiety problems [Zahn-Waxler, Shirtcliff & Marceau, 2008].

Issues, Conundrums and Questions: Why This Is Harder than You Might Think

Although some developmental scientists perceive biological measures as objective and concrete, even something as 'basic' as a change in heart rate can be produced by numerous processes, and the functional significance of that change varies depending on the origin of the change. The appropriate implementation of physiological indices into studies of emotional development, combined with careful consideration of the data they produce, can bring new levels of understanding to the field. We stress *appropriate* and *careful*, because the perplexing issues that regularly pose challenges for developmental research also raise their thorny heads for the study of developmental affective psychophysiology, with extras tossed in for good measure [e.g., Dennis et al., 2012, 2013]. We emphasize a particular subset of problems that need to be kept in mind while evaluating existing research, and which serve to inform next steps for future studies.

What Is the Essential Nature of Emotions?

A long-standing debate among emotion theorists is whether early emotions are evident as quantitative variations along dimensions, such as activation and valence [Lindquist & Barrett, 2008], or as discrete or basic categories, like anger or fear [Izard, 2007]. Closely connected to this, two perennial debates in emotional psychophysiology are whether discrete emotions are distinguishable at the biological level, and whether there is specificity of association between a given physiological measure and a given emotional construct [Dennis et al., 2012]. Some meta-analyses and multi-measure studies suggest that examining patterns across several autonomic physiological measures reveals consistent differences between such basic emotions as sadness, fear, anger, disgust, and happiness [Rainville, Bechara, Naqvi & Damasio, 2006; Stemmler, 2004]. Others contest these conclusions, arguing that the data are more congruent with dimensional or constructionist models. Even recent meta-analyses of neuroimaging research on emotion and brain activity have failed to resolve this debate, both providing support for discrete emotions theory and the distinctiveness of basic emotions in terms of regions and patterns of neural activation [Vytal & Hamann, 2010], and failing to find such distinct patterns, consistent with constructionist theory [Lindquist, Wager, Kober, Bliss-Moreau & Barrett, 2012]. While the interpretation of meta-analytic evidence can be biased by *a priori* theoretical frameworks [Buck, 2012; Caruana & Gallese, 2012], the lack of definitive answers fuels ongoing debate about the essential nature of emotion.

What Develops in the Physiology of Emotions?

Studying any aspect of development is like trying to get hold of a moving target. The challenge is at least trebled in developmental affective psychophysiology: physiological systems are developing, emotions are developing, and the relations between physiology and emotions also are developing. Adding further complexity, the multicomponent nature of emotion includes the multiple levels of physiological activity that have been linked to emotion. These multiple physiological systems are mutually influential and share bidirectional paths of communication; the connections between these systems change over development, and the contributions that these systems make to emotion and development are integrated, coordinated and dynamic [Larsen, Berntson, Poehlmann, Ito & Cacioppo, 2008; Miskovic & Schmidt, 2012]. Developmental scientists have begun to examine the associations between emotion constructs and the interactive and systemic effects of multiple physiological measures, particularly in the areas of temperament and emotional problems [El-Sheikh et al., 2009; Furtunato, Dribin, Granger & Buss, 2008]. However, most of what is known about emotions and the integration of CNS, HPA, hypothalamic-pituitary-gonadal axis, ANS and skeletomotor activity is based on research with adults. We do not know how maturation and experience influence the development of top-down regulation of peripheral affective physiology, or bottom-up influences on central emotional processing. The peripheral, hormonal, neural, cognitive, and behavioral aspects of emotion mature and change over time, and they continually influence each other. The challenge for emotion researchers, then, is to determine whether and how earlier changes in one physiological system or level support development in others.

What Is the Role of Time in Developmental Affective Psychophysiology?

Efforts to examine the chronometry of physiological changes associated with emotions confront numerous challenges [Fox et al., 2012]. Emotions vary in their temporal features, such as onset and duration. How to distinguish emotion from emotion regulation, or how to recognize when top-down or bottom-up regulatory influences are affecting the physiology of an elicited emotional response, remains uncertain. For example, when is the off-set, or recovery period, of an emotion a product of that emotion's temporal features, and when is it the result of regulatory efforts to maintain or foreshorten the affective experience?

All stages of the research process – design, measurement, and analysis – require accounting for time. Establishing and identifying the appropriate baseline, comparison condition, or starting point for the initiation of an emotional process is not straightforward, and obtaining repeated measurements is required to examine the changes that occur over the course of the emotion [Obradović & Boyce, 2012]. The appropriate units of time for sampling – milliseconds, seconds, minutes or longer – also vary depending on the physiological index (e.g., ERP versus RSA) and emotional construct (e.g., facial expression versus mood) being examined. For many physiological measures, standardized parameters have yet to be established for optimal sampling periods, and descriptive developmental research has not identified age-based parameters. Moreover, researchers are still developing appropriate statistical models to capture patterns of change over the multiple associated components of emotion [Brooker & Buss, 2010; Burt & Obradović, 2013; Helm, Sbarra & Ferrer, 2012]. Finally, the temporal features of emotion cannot be assumed to generalize across development. What is typical or adaptive for the course of emotional physiology might differ for infants, children, youths and adults.

What Is the Role of Context in Developmental Affective Psychophysiology?

Emotion and emotion regulation are contextually bound. Their meanings and implications for functioning must be understood in relation to the context within which they occur. For example, how we interpret a child's excitement and laughter differs depending on whether that child is at a puppet show or is watching a fight on the playground, and on whether the child is 5 or 15 years old. Across situations and ages, phenotypically identical behaviors can arise from different physiological substrates. The contexts of emotional physiology are also shaped by children's past histories, social relationships, and individual goals. Developmental researchers have not yet made a concerted effort in determining how context can be quantified and incorporated into studies of emotional physiology.

How Does the Interplay of Nature and Nurture Shape Affective Psychophysiology?

Researchers now commonly recognize that any measure of physiological activity cannot be presumed to reflect 'nature', 'genetics', or some other singular point of origin. The field of epigenetics is focused on identifying how experiential factors influence gene activity, thereby contributing to biological functioning and behavioral expression. There is strong evidence that life experiences, including relationships with caregivers, contribute to the development of the physiological systems involved in emotion [Feldman, 2012b; Strang et al., 2012]. Initially, regulation of the emotional distress of infants is primarily the responsibility of caregivers, with the ability to self-regulate increasing over the first years of life. Scientists are just beginning to understand how external regulation experiences shape the diverse aspects of physiological capacities for self-regulation [Henderson & Mundy, 2013]. We know even less about whether and how children's emotional physiology relates to interactions with peers and involvement with cultural norms and values, as well as the degree to which it can be influenced by socioeconomic conditions or exposure to environmental stimuli [see Ellis, Boyce, Belsky, Bakermans-Kranenburg & Van IJzendoorn, 2011]. Developmental psychologists continue to formulate unified theories that incorporate the transactional or dialectical influences of nature and nurture on development [Sameroff, 2010], and researchers interested in the intersections of development, physiology, and emotion similarly need to recognize the multiple and complex origins for the phenomena they study.

Should We Examine Central Tendencies or Individual Differences?

Given the diversity, complexity, and nuance involved in studying developmental affective psychophysiology, efforts to identify the 'typical' or 'average' links between physiology and emotion at given points of development might be misguided. Just as the average high temperature for the month of July might be 80°F (or 26°C) without any of its 31 days actually having a high of 80°F, so too might a mean change in heart rate associated with a mean intensity of fearful expression fail to accurately describe the heart and face of any given child. One reason why efforts to find emotion-specific physiology often produce small effect sizes or failures to replicate could be that individual differences overwhelm central tendencies. Studies of temperament and emotional problems inherently involve examinations of individual differences. Associations between physiology and state emotions, as assessed through reported feelings or observed facial expressions, can differ greatly for children with varying traits, such as inhibited versus uninhibited temperaments [Theall-Honey & Schmidt, 2006], or clinical versus normative levels of disruptive behaviors [Marsh, Beauchaine & Williams, 2008]. Conversely, when researchers have the goal of measuring typical or average aspects of emotional physiology, individual differences can be overlooked or seen merely as contributing noise or measurement error to the data.

This is not to argue that there is no value in efforts to measure central tendencies. To know how emotional processes should be expected to change over development, we need to know typical parameters at given ages. To identify when a child's emotional functioning warrants intervention, we must have a sense of what is healthy functioning. At the same time, this work should be pursued with the expectation that there might be a broad window of expectable and healthy emotional physiology at any given age, in any given environment, and that variations in the patterns of association among components of emotion are themselves meaningful and informative.

Wading Into the Choppy Seas: Our Recent Work on Developmental Affective Psychophysiology

Our own recent studies of emotional physiology in children and adolescents have been directed toward tackling the conundrums and questions described in the preceding section. We do not pretend to have solved these enduring riddles. We hope, though, that our approaches and findings will inform the ongoing discussions and spark further investigation.

Specificity, Central Tendencies, and Individual Differences

The multiple components of an emotional response need to be coordinated in order to motivate appropriate motor action patterns to deal with evoking stimuli [Levenson, 1994]. Thus, for emotions to be functional as regulating processes, the components of emotion should be coherent. In a large sample of adolescents over-represented for emotional and behavioral problems, we used hierarchical linear modeling to examine the coherence of heart rate changes and subjective feelings (intensity of self-reported emotions) in response to videotaped scenes targeted to elicit sadness, fear, anger, and happiness [Hastings et al., 2009]. Within youths, there was evidence for coherence of sadness and fear: Youths who reported more intense fear had higher heart rates than those who felt less fear (appropriate for escape/avoidance), whereas the intensity of sadness was inversely associated with heart rate (appropriate for surrender/seeking help). We documented even greater variation in patterns of coherence across youths, though. For example, the cardiac arousal of youths with clinical levels of externalizing problems was unrelated to the intensity of their feelings. These data suggest that although such youths may have *felt* frightened by scary scenes or saddened by others' distress, they lacked the corresponding cardiac arousal that would have prepared them to display typically-expected actions to cope with the eliciting situation. This fits with research characterizing disruptive and aggressive youths as fearless and lacking sympathy or empathic sadness [Beauchaine, 2012; Zahn-Waxler et al., 2008].

Adding Time and Mechanism

Heart rate changes can serve as useful indices of overall arousal; however, they do not reveal which neurobiological systems caused the changes. According to Polyvagal theory, dynamic changes in RSA are important for regulating emotional arousal. Many studies of RSA and emotion have failed to adequately capture the dynamic time-course of emotions and emotion regulation in their analyses. Examining change as a static index, such as a difference score between baseline and emotional conditions, presumes change is linear and overlooks fluctuations within conditions [Burt & Obradović, 2013]. Using repeated measurements, we have studied PNS regulation using latent growth curve (LGC) modeling to examine nonlinear slopes of RSA change in response to emotion inductions. We showed young children the Mood Induction Stimulus for Children (MISC) [Zahn-Waxler, Cole, Welsh & Fox, 1995], and sampled RSA over a 60-second anger story that involved four narrated pictures, each presented for 15 s [Miller et al., 2013a]. On average, children exhibited RSA suppression from (1) the neutral introduction to (2) the initiation of anger. This was followed by RSA augmentation (or rebound) in (3) the intensification of anger, and stable RSA through (4) the mildly positive resolution. LGC analyses revealed a significant latent basis slope of nonlinear change that fit the RSA data better than linear or quadratic models. Thus, children's PNS response to the anger story was first to withdraw vagal influence on cardiac activity, which could have supported increased attention to the stimulus and preparedness to act, followed by application of the vagal brake, which could have helped children to keep calm and still while watching the story unfold.

Variability in this typical pattern of nonlinear change also had functional significance. Experimenters interviewed children about their aggressive responses to provocations by peers. Children with stronger latent slopes – more suppression followed by more augmentation – reported less aggression than youths with weaker slopes. On their own, examined as change scores, neither RSA suppression nor RSA augmentation predicted aggression. Girls and older children also had stronger slopes than boys and younger children, respectively, consistent with gender and age differences in the regulation of anger and aggression [Card, Stucky, Sawalani & Little, 2008; Lemerise & Dodge, 2008]. We interpret these findings as showing that better parasympathetic regulation of anger is evidenced by nonlinear RSA change over the course of an anger episode.

But is parasympathetic regulation of anger characteristic of other emotional contexts? The MISC also included sad stories that followed the same temporal structure as the anger one. Children's RSA showed a similar pattern of suppression, followed by augmentation, then stability, which was again best fit in LGC modeling by a latent basis slope [Miller, Nuselovici, Chochol & Hastings, 2013b]. This nonlinear latent slope predicted children's displays of empathic concern in response to adults' simulations of pain and distress. Unlike the anger analyses, though, the change score of RSA augmentation during the intensely sad portion of the story (segment 3) also was uniquely associated with empathic concern, suggesting that PNS support for calm engagement while viewing others' sadness might facilitate children's preparedness to act on their behalf [Hastings & Miller, in press]. In support of trait perspectives on emotion regulation, the latent slopes for anger and for sadness were correlated: Children showed similar patterns of RSA change across the emotional contexts. In support of emotion-specific physiology, the latent slope of RSA during sadness did not predict control of aggressive impulses, and the latent slope of RSA during anger did not predict empathic concern. Thus, on the question of whether emotion regulation in children should be considered a matter of 'being well-regulated' or of 'regulating well,' these data lend support for the importance of both trait and state emotional physiology.

Considering Context, Extending Time, and Adding Levels

Although researchers commonly use pictures and videos to induce emotions in psychophysiology research, such methods arguably lack ecological validity. That is, there could be striking differences in children's emotional physiology for scenes they observe versus events they experience. As well, when real-world events provoke emotional arousal, part of regulation involves recovering from the event. There has been little developmental work on recovery from physiological reactivity. Moreover, even though examining RSA provides more neurobiological specificity than examining heart rate, the PNS is just one branch of the ANS.

In some of our current work [Kahle, Lopez, Miller & Hastings, 2013], we examined changes in PNS (using RSA) and SNS (using PEP) during 3 1/2-year-old children's reactivity to and recovery from a frustratingly impossible task: Being asked to draw a perfect green circle [from LabTAB; Goldsmith & Rothbart, 1996]. RSA and PEP were sampled 10 times through the 3-min frustrating task (task) and 3 times in the subsequent 1 min during which the examiner praised the child's efforts (recovery). A multi-phase LGC approach allowed the estimation of separate slopes for task and recovery. Changes in PEP were linear, with PEP shortening across the task (increasing SNS influence) and lengthening in recovery (decreasing SNS influence). A latent basis model fit the RSA data well because change was nonlinear. After almost a minute of no change, RSA began to decrease (less PNS influence). This decrease in RSA continued through the recovery period. Thus, the task physiology could be characterized initially as coactivity, but as reciprocal sympathetic activation once PNS influence begins to withdraw, consistent with anger or stress responses. The recovery period could be characterized as autonomic co-inhibition, with lessening cardiac innervation from both ANS branches [Berntson et al., 2007].

Results also revealed significant variability around the slopes. Mothers reported on children's concurrent trait emotion regulation. Only the PEP recovery slope was associated with emotion regulation. Children who had stronger decreases in sympathetic innervation during recovery were described as more emotionally well-regulated. Phrased the other way, children who were seen by their mothers as less well-regulated maintained a pattern of sympathetic activation, akin to a fight-or-flight response, for longer after the examiner ended the provocation and tried to induce a positive mood. Therefore, although SNS activation is normatively expected when one experiences a frustrating event, it might be the swift termination of this activity when a frustrating situation has been resolved that distinguishes children who are characterized as emotionally well-regulated from their less well-regulated peers.

Looking at Socialization and Development

Finally, many of our studies have included considerations of parental socialization styles and practices in relation to children's physiology and emotion. Paralleling others [Feldman, 2012b; Katz & Rigterink, 2012], we have seen some evidence that socialization contributes to the development of emotional physiology in toddlers and preschoolers. Longitudinal analyses showed that earlier negative control by mothers and fathers predict less RSA augmentation, or more suppression, during play with peers [Hastings, Nuselovici et al., 2008]. Children with greater RSA augmentation had fewer emotional problems and better self-regulatory behaviors, and their RSA during peer play mediated associations between maternal negative control and children's adjustment. As well, we have linked maternal negative control to preschoolers' cortisol reactivity in response to meeting adult strangers [Hastings et al., 2011]. Polyvagal theory links higher RSA with preparedness for more calm social engagement, and elevated HPA reactivity reflects stress from perceived threats to self. Thus, these findings suggest that aversive parenting practices, which impair the development of emotional competence [Cicchetti et al., this volume; Denham, Bassett & Wyatt, 2007], might contribute to maladjustment by undermining the adaptive functioning of children's emotional physiology.

We have also found that maternal and paternal socialization moderates associations between physiology and children's emotional functioning. Some findings have been in accord with the differential susceptibility to environment model [Ellis et al., 2011], such that children with a particular pattern of emotional physiology displayed adjustment that was worse or better than average depending on their experience of more aversive or supportive socialization. Low basal RSA, less RSA suppression to a cognitive challenge, and greater cortisol reactivity to a social stressor could all be considered markers of sensitivity or susceptibility. We found that children with low (but not high) basal RSA had few internalizing problems if fathers avoided being either dismissive or exaggerating of children's negative emotions, but elevated internalizing problems if fathers used such emotion socialization techniques [Hastings & De, 2008]. Similarly, children who evidenced less (but not more) RSA suppression had few internalizing problems if fathers were warm and supportive during dyadic interactions, but elevated problems if fathers showed little positive engagement [Hastings, Sullivan et al., 2008]. In addition, we found that preschool-aged boys with elevated HPA reactivity were most susceptible to mothers' angry, punitive behaviors. Concurrently, they had fewer or more externalizing problems than less reactive boys if mothers avoided versus relied upon such aversive practices, respectively [Hastings et al., 2011].

The differential susceptibilities model turns our earlier consideration of context on its head. In effect, children's patterns of emotional physiology might serve as the context in which socialization influences development. Children process and internalize the experiences they have with their caregivers, constructing schemas and values that shape how they engage with their broadening social worlds over development. Their interpretations of and accommodations to these socialization experiences, however, differ depending on children's neurobiological reactivity and regulation. Not all of our interaction effects have fit neatly into the differential susceptibilities model, with some appearing to be more in accord with diathesis-stress or organismic specificity models [e.g., Miller et al., 2013a]. Still, these and other such frameworks for explaining and examining transactional biopsychosocial processes [e.g., Del Giudice, Ellis & Shirtcliff, 2011; Sameroff, 2010] hold great promise for advancing research on developmental affective psychophysiology.

Moving Forward

At the 2003 Emotions and Emotional Development Preconference, held in Tampa Florida at the Biennial Meeting of the Society for Research in Child Development, attendees sat at several small tables for break-out discussions on numerous topics of 'Emotions and…': socialization influences, gender differences, emotion regulation, etc. When the time came to share, at table after table, the chosen spokesperson related the challenges vexing that group of developmental scientists, and ended by saying 'And we think that adding measures of physiology might add some clarity to this'. That continued until the spokesperson from the 'emotion and physiology' table stood and said, basically, 'Don't hold your breath'.

After a decade of advances in theory, technology and research, a different response would be warranted today. Developmental scientists are formulating integrative, multilevel models of emotional development that incorporate time, contexts, relationships, and individual differences. We are evaluating these models with well-designed studies, careful measurement, innovative analyses and insightful interpretations of their findings. Although there is much to be learned, we now have a better array of techniques and expertise, and a solid conceptual and empirical basis from which we can launch the next generation of studies on development, emotions, and physiology. The vexing challenges that have been perennial issues in this field have not gotten any easier, but we are closer now to addressing them directly. The fledgling science of developmental affective psychophysiology has matured, and the next decade stands to be an even more exciting period of discovery.

Acknowledgements

The research described in this report was conducted with the support of the NIMH Intramural Program, the Canadian Institutes of Health Research, the Fetzer Institute, and Graduate Research Fellowships from the National Science Foundation awarded to the second and third authors.

References

Adam, E.K. (2012). Emotion-cortisol transactions occur over multiple time scales in development: Implications for research on emotion and the development of emotional disorders. *Monographs of the Society for Research in Child Development, 77*, 79–86.

Barrett, K.C., Fox, N.A., Morgan, G.A., Fidler, D.J., & Daunhauer, L.A. (Eds.). (2013). *Handbook of self-regulatory processes in development: New directions and international perspectives.* New York: Psychology Press.

Beauchaine, T.P. (2001). Vagal tone, development, and Gray's motivational theory: Toward an integrated model of autonomic nervous system functioning in psychopathology. *Development and Psychopathology, 13*, 183–214.

Beauchaine, T.P. (2012). Physiological markers of emotion and behavior dysregulation in externalizing psychopathology. *Monographs of the Society for Research in Child Development, 77*, 79–86.

Berntson, G., & Cacioppo, J. (2007). Integrative physiology: Homeostasis, allostasis, and the orchestration of systemic physiology. In J.T. Cacioppo, L.G. Tassinary & G. Berntson (Eds.), *Handbook of psychophysiology* (2nd ed., pp. 433–452). New York: Cambridge University Press.

Berntson, G.G., Quigley, K.S., & Lozano, D. (2007). Cardiovascular psychophysiology. In J.T. Cacioppo, L.G. Tassinary & G. Berntson (Eds.), *Handbook of psychophysiology* (2nd ed., pp. 182–210). New York: Cambridge University Press.

Bradley, M.M., & Lang, P.J. (2007). Emotion and motivation. In J.T. Cacioppo, L.G. Tassinary & G. Berntson (Eds.), *Handbook of psychophysiology* (2nd ed., pp. 581–607). New York: Cambridge University Press.

Brooker, R.J., & Buss, K.A. (2010). Dynamic measures of RSA predict distress and regulation in toddlers. *Developmental Psychobiology, 52*, 372–382.

Buck, R.W. (2012). Prime elements of subjectively experienced feelings and desires: Imaging the emotional cocktail. *The Behavioral and Brain Sciences, 35*, 144.

Burt, K.B., & Obradović, J. (2013). The construct of psychophysiological reactivity: Statistical and psychometric issues. *Developmental Review, 33*, 29–57.

Card, N.A., Stucky, B.D., Sawalani, G.M., Little, T.D. (2008). Direct and indirect aggression during childhood and adolescence: A meta-analytic review of gender differences, intercorrelations, and relations to maladjustment. *Child Development, 79,* 1185–1229.

Caruana, F., & Gallese, V. (2012). Overcoming the emotion experience/expression dichotomy. *Behavioral and Brain Sciences, 35*, 145–146.

Casey, B.J., Getz, S., & Galvan, A. (2008). The adolescent brain. *Developmental Review, 28*, 62–77.

Cole, P.M., Martin, S.E., & Dennis, T.A. (2004). Emotion regulation as a scientific construct: Methodological challenges and directions for child development research. *Child Development, 75*, 317–333.

Critchley, H.D. (2005). Neural mechanisms of autonomic, affective, and cognitive integration. *The Journal of Comparative Neurology, 493*, 154–166.

Decety, J., & Michalska, K.J. (2010). Neurodevelopmental changes in the circuits underlying empathy and sympathy from childhood to adulthood. *Developmental Science, 13*, 886–899.

DeCicco, J.M., Solomon, B., & Dennis, T.A. (2012). Neural correlates of cognitive reappraisal in children: An ERP study. *Developmental Cognitive Neuroscience, 2*, 70–80.

Del Giudice, M., Ellis, B.J., & Shirtcliff, E.A. (2011). The adaptive calibration model of stress responsivity. *Neuroscience & Biobehavioral Reviews, 35*, 1562–1592.

Denham, S.A., Bassett, H.H., & Wyatt, T. (2007). The socialization of emotional competence. In P.D. Hastings & J.E. Grusec (Eds.), *Handbook of socialization: Theory and research* (pp. 614–637). New York: Guilford Press.

Dennis, T.A., Buss, K.A., & Hastings, P.D. (Eds.). (2012). Introduction to the Monograph: Physiological measures of emotion from a developmental perspective: State of the science. *Monographs of the Society for Research in Child Development, 77*, 1–5.

Dennis, T.A., O'Toole, L.J., & DeCicco, J.M. (2013). Emotion regulation from the perspective of developmental neuroscience: What, where, when, and why. In K.C. Barrett, N.A. Fox, G.A. Morgan, D.J. Fidler & L.A. Daunhauer (Eds.), *Handbook of self-regulatory processes in development: New directions and international perspectives* (pp. 135–172). New York: Psychology Press.

de Veld, D.M.J., Riksen-Walraven, J.M., & de Weerth, C. (2012). The relation between emotion regulation strategies and physiological stress responses in middle childhood. *Psychoneuroendocrinology, 37*, 1309–1319.

Ellis, B.J., Boyce, W.T., Belsky, J., Bakermans-Kranenburg, M.J., & Van IJzendoorn, M.H. (2011). Differential susceptibility to the environment: An evolutionary-neurodevelopmental theory. *Development and Psychopathology, 23*, 7–28.

El-Sheikh, M., Kouros, C.D., Erath, S., Cummings, E.M., Keller, P., & Staton, L. (2009). Marital conflict and children's externalizing behavior: Pathways involving interactions between parasympathetic and sympathetic nervous system activity. *Monographs of the Society for Research in Child Development, 74.*

Feldman, R. (2012a). Oxytocin and social affiliation in humans. *Hormones and Behavior, 61*, 380–391.

Feldman, R. (2012b). Parent-infant synchrony: A biobehavioral model of mutual influences in the formation of affiliative bonds. *Monographs of the Society for Research in Child Development, 77*, 42–51.

Fortunato, C.K., Dribin, A.E., Granger, D.A., & Buss, K.A. (2008). Salivary alpha-amylase and cortisol in toddlers: Differential relations to affective behavior. *Developmental Psychobiology, 50*, 807–818.

Fowles, D.C. (1988). Psychophysiology and psychopathology: A motivational approach. *Psychophysiology, 25*, 373–391.

Fox, N.A., Kirwan, M., & Reeb-Sutherland, B. (2012). Measuring the physiology of emotion and emotion regulation – Timing is everything. *Monographs of the Society for Research in Child Development, 77*, 98–108.

Giedd, J.N., & Rapoport, J.L. (2010). Structural MRI of pediatric brain development: What have we learned and where are we going? *Neuron, 67*, 728–734.

Goldsmith, H.H., & Rothbart, M. (1996). *The laboratory temperament assessment battery manual.* Madison: Personality Development Laboratory, University of Wisconsin.

Gullone, E., Hughes, E.K., King, N.J., & Tonge, B. (2010). The normative development of emotion regulation strategy use in children and adolescents: A 2-year follow-up study. *Journal of Child Psychology and Psychiatry, 51*, 567–574.

Gunnar, M.R., & Adam, E.K. (2012). The hypothalamic-pituitary-adrenocortical system and emotion: Current wisdom and future directions. *Monographs of the Society for Research in Child Development, 77*, 109–119.

Hastings, P.D., & De, I. (2008). Parasympathetic regulation and parental socialization of emotion: Biopsychosocial processes of adjustment in preschoolers. *Social Development, 17*, 211–238.

Hastings, P.D., & Miller, J.G. (In Press). Autonomic regulation, Polyvagal Theory, and children's prosocial development. In L. Padilla-Walker & G. Carlo (Eds.), *The multidimensionality of prosocial behavior: Biological, socialization, and contextual perspectives.* New York: Oxford University Press.

Hastings, P.D., Miller, J.G., Kahle, S., & Zahn-Waxler, C. (2014). The neurobiological bases of empathic concern for others. In M. Killen & J. Smetana (Eds.), *Handbook of moral development, 2nd ed.* (pp. 411–434) New Jersey, Lawrence Erlbaum.

Hastings, P.D., Nuselovici, J.N., Klimes-Dougan, B., Kendziora, K.T., Usher, B.A., Ho, M.R., & Zahn-Waxler, C. (2009). Dysregulated coherence of subjective and cardiac emotional activation in adolescents with internalizing and externalizing problems. *Journal of Child Psychology and Psychiatry, 50*, 1348–1356.

Hastings, P.D., Nuselovici, J.N., Utendale, W.T., Coutya, J., McShane, K.E., & Sullivan, C. (2008). Applying the polyvagal theory to children's emotion regulation: Social context, socialization, and adjustment. *Biological Psychology, 79*, 299–306.

Hastings, P.D., Ruttle, P.L., Serbin, L.A., Mills, R.S.L., Stack, D.M., & Schwartzman, A.E. (2011). Adrenocortical responses to strangers in preschoolers: Relations with parenting, temperament, and psychopathology. *Developmental Psychobiology, 53*, 694–710.

Hastings, P.D., Sullivan, C., McShane, K.E., Coplan, R.J., Utendale, W.T., & Vyncke, J.D. (2008). Parental socialization, vagal regulation, and preschoolers' anxious difficulties: Direct mothers and moderated fathers. *Child Development, 79*, 45–64.

Helm, J.L., Sbarra, D., & Ferrer, E. (2012). Assessing cross-partner associations in physiological responses via coupled oscillator models. *Emotion, 12*, 748–762.

Henderson, H.A., & Mundy, P.C. (2013). The integration of self and other in the development of self-regulation: Typical and atypical processes. In K.C. Barrett, N.A. Fox, G.A. Morgan, D.J. Fidler & L.A. Daunhauer (Eds.), *Handbook of self-regulatory processes in development: New directions and international perspectives* (pp. 113–134). New York: Psychology Press.

Izard, C.E. (2007). Basic emotions, natural kinds, emotion schemas, and a new paradigm. *Perspectives on Psychological Science, 2*, 260–280.

Kahle, S., Lopez, M., Miller, J., Hastings, P.D. (April, 2013). The role of autonomic recovery in the development of emotion regulation. Paper presented at the biannual meeting of the *Society for Research in Child Development*, Seattle.

Kaltas, G.A., & Chrousos, G.P. (2007). The neuroendocrinology of stress. In J.T. Cacioppo, L.G. Tassinary & G.C. Bernston (Eds.), *Handbook of psychophysiology* (2nd ed., pp. 303–318). New York: Cambridge University Press.

Katz, L.F., & Rigterink, T. (2012). Domestic violence and emotion socialization. *Monographs of the Society for Research in Child Development, 77*, 52–60.

Larsen, J.T., Berntson, G.G., Poehlhmann, K.M., Ito, T.A., & Cacioppo, J.T. (2008). The psychophysiology of emotion. In M. Lewis, J.M. Haviland-Jones & L.F. Barrett (Eds.), *Handbook of emotions* (3rd ed., pp. 180–195). New York: Guilford.

Lemerise, E.A., & Dodge, K.A. (2008). The development of anger and hostile interactions. In M. Lewis, J.M. Haviland-Jones & L.F. Barrett (Eds.), *Handbook of emotions* (3rd ed., pp. 730–741). New York: Guilford.

Levenson, R.W. (1994). Human emotions: A functional view. In P. Ekman & R.J. Davidson (Eds.), *The nature of emotion: Fundamental questions* (pp. 123–126). New York: Oxford University Press.

Lindquist, K.A., & Barrett, L.F. (2008). Emotional complexity. In M. Lewis, J.M. Haviland-Jones & L.F. Barrett (Eds.), *Handbook of emotions* (3rd ed., pp. 513–530). New York: Guilford.

Lindquist, K.A., Wager, T.D., Kober, H., Bliss-Moreau, E., & Barrett, L.F. (2012). The brain basis of emotion: A meta-analytic review. *The Behavioral and Brain Sciences, 35*, 121–143.

Madsen, K.S., Baare, W.F.F., Vestergaard, M., Skimminge, A., Ejersbo, L.R., Ramsøy, T.Z., & Jernigan, T.L. (2010). Response inhibition is associated with white matter microstructure in children. *Neuropsychologia, 48*, 854–862.

Marcovitch, S., Leigh, J., Calkins, S.D., Leerks, E.M., O'Brien, M., & Blankson, A.N. (2010). Moderate vagal withdrawal in 3.5-year-old children is associated with optimal performance on executive function tasks. *Developmental Psychobiology, 52*, 603–608.

Marsh, P., Beauchaine, T.P., & Williams, B. (2008). Dissociation of sad facial expression and autonomic nervous system responding in boys with disruptive behavior disorders. *Psychophysiology, 45*, 100–110.

Miller, J.G., Chocol, C., Nuselovici, J.N., Utendale, W.T., Simard, M., & Hastings, P.D. (2013a). Children's dynamic RSA change during anger and its relations with parenting, temperament, and control of aggression. *Biological Psychology, 92*, 417–425.

Miller, J.G., Nuselovici, J., Chochol, C., & Hastings, P.D. (2013b). Dynamic changes in RSA during sadness predict the development of empathy. Paper presented at the *Biennial Meeting of the Society for Research in Child Development*. Seattle.

Mills, R.S.L., Imm, G.P., Walling, B.R., & Weiler, H.A. (2008). Cortisol reactivity and regulation associated with shame responding in early childhood. *Developmental Psychology, 44*, 1369–1380.

Miskovic, V., & Schmidt, L.A. (2012). New directions in the study of individual differences in temperament: A brain-body approach to understanding fearful and fearless children. *Monographs of the Society for Research in Child Development, 77*, 28–38.

Murphy, F.C., Nimmo-Smith, I., & Lawrence, A.D. (2003). Functional neuroanatomy of emotions: A meta-analysis. *Cognitive, Affective, & Behavioral Neuroscience, 3*, 207–233.

Obradović, J., & Boyce, W.T. (2012). Developmental psychophysiology of emotion processes. *Monographs of the Society for Research in Child Development, 77*, 120–128.

Perlman, S.B., & Pelphrey, K.A. (2011). Developing connections for affective regulation: Age-related changes in emotional brain connectivity. *Journal of Experimental Child Psychology, 108*, 607–620.

Perry, N.B., Calkins, S.D., Nelson, J.A., Leerkes, E.M., & Marcovitch, S. (2012). Mothers' responses to children's negative emotions and child emotion regulation: The moderating role of vagal suppression. *Developmental Psychobiology, 54*, 503–513.

Porges, S.W. (2007). The polyvagal perspective. *Biological Psychology, 74*, 116–143.

Rainville, P., Bechara, A., Naqvi, N., & Damasio, A.R. (2006). Basic emotions are associated with distinct patterns of cardiovascular reactivity. *International Journal of Psychophysiology, 61*, 5–18.

Rutter, M., & Sroufe, L.A. (2000). Developmental psychopathology: Concepts and challenges. *Development and Psychopathology, 12*, 265–296.

Sameroff, A. (2010). A unified theory of development: A dialectic integration of nature and nurture. *Child Development, 81*, 6–22.

Schmitz, A., Merikangas, K., Swendsen, H., Cui, L., Heaton, L., & Grillon, C. (2011). Measuring anxious responses to predictable and unpredictable threat in children and adolescents. *Journal of Experimental Child Psychology, 110*, 159–170.

Shiner, R.L., Buss, K.A., McClowry, S.G., Putnam, S.P., Saudino, K.J., & Zentner, M. (2012). What is temperament now? Assessing progress in temperament research on the twenty-fifth anniversary of Goldsmith et al. (1987). *Child Development Perspectives, 6*, 436–444.

Strang, N.M., Hanson, J.L., & Pollak, S.D. (2012). The importance of biological methods in linking social experience with social and emotional development. *Monographs of the Society for Research in Child Development, 77*, 61–66.

Stemmler, G. (2004). Physiological processes during emotion. In P. Philippot & R.S. Feldman (Eds.), *The regulation of emotion* (pp. 33–70) Mahwah: Lawrence Erlbaum Associates.

Tassinary, L.G., Cacioppo, J.T., & Vanman, E.J. (2007). The skeletomotor system: Surface electromyography. In J.T. Cacioppo, L.G. Tassinary & G. Berntson (Eds.), *Handbook of psychophysiology* (2nd ed., pp. 267–302). New York: Cambridge University Press.

Theall-Honey, L., & Schmidt, L. (2006). Do temperamentally shy children process emotion differently than nonshy children? Behavioral, psychophysiological, and gender differences in reticent preschoolers. *Developmental Psychobiology, 48*, 187–196.

Thompson, R.A. (2011a). Methods and measures in developmental emotions research: Some assembly required. *Journal of Experimental Child Psychology, 110*, 275–285.

Thompson, R.A. (2011b). Emotion and emotion regulation: Two sides of the developing coin. *Emotion Review, 3*, 53–61.

Vytal, K., & Hamann, S. (2010). Neuroimaging support for discrete neural correlates of basic emotions: A voxel-based meta-analysis. *Journal of Cognitive Neuroscience, 22*, 2864–2885.

Zahn-Waxler, C., Cole, P.M., Welsh, J.D., & Fox, N.A. (1995). Psychophysiological correlates of empathy and prosocial behaviors in preschool children with behavior problems. *Development and Psychopathology, 7*, 27–48.

Zahn-Waxler, C., Shirtcliff, E.A., & Marceau, K. (2008). Disorders of childhood and adolescence: Gender and psychopathology. *Annual Review of Clinical Psychology, 4*, 275–303.

Paul D. Hastings
Department of Psychology, University of California Davis
One Shields Ave
Davis CA 95616 (USA)
E-Mail pdhastings@ucdavis.edu

Hansen Lagattuta K (ed): Children and Emotion. New Insights into Developmental Affective Sciences.
Contrib Hum Dev. Basel, Karger, 2014, vol 26, pp 29–41 (DOI: 10.1159/000354349)

Emotional Development in Maltreated Children

Dante Cicchetti[a, b] · Rowena Ng[a]

[a]Institute of Child Development, University of Minnesota, Minneapolis, Minn., [b]Mt. Hope Family Center, University of Rochester, Rochester, Minn., USA

Abstract

Child maltreatment represents one of the most adverse and stressful challenges that confront children. As the maltreating home is a dramatic violation of environments believed to promote adaptive and healthy development, research on child maltreatment informs developmental theory by elucidating the conditions necessary for normal emotional development. Maltreated children are exposed to an atypical emotional climate, characterized by less positive and more negative emotions than are generally expressed in nonmaltreating families. These aberrant emotional experiences can eventuate in neuropathological connections that undermine effective perception, regulation, processing, and understanding of emotions. Future directions in research on maltreatment and emotional development are discussed, including implications for implementing and evaluating preventive interventions.

The empirical investigation of the emotions possesses obvious importance for comprehending the processes underlying atypical development. One of the consequences of examining normal emotional processes is that this underscores the criticality of constructing a theoretical model of the ontogenesis of the emotions that can distinguish between well-adjusted and maladaptive emotional development. Historically, developmentalists have stressed the importance of studying atypical or psychopathological development in the formulation of a comprehensive developmental theory [Cicchetti, 1990; Kaplan, 1966]. Clinicians and researchers who have studied an array of mental disorders, including autism, depression, bipolar disorder, psychopathy, and schizophrenia [Cicchetti, Ackerman & Izard, 1995], have stressed the emotional as well as the cognitive and biological aspects of the ontogenesis of psychopathology.

Research investigations of the emotions in atypical populations can enhance our understanding of the processes involved in normal emotional development [Hesse & Cicchetti, 1982]. To theorize about emotional development without a consideration of the deviations that might be expected from prominent and pervasive intra- and extra-organismic disturbances, as well as the transactions among them, would result in an incomplete and ambiguous portrayal of the developmental process [Cicchetti & Schneider-Rosen, 1984]. Consistent with a developmental psychopathology perspective, the examination of maladaptive and psychopathological development can help to elucidate the mechanisms of normal development [Cicchetti, 1984, 1993; Rutter, 1986; Sroufe, 1990]. In typical development, the component developmental systems may be so well integrated that it is difficult to determine how normal functioning depends on this integration. When there is an obvious perturbation or disturbance in a component system, an examination of how that atypicality relates to the organization of other component systems can reveal important information regarding the interdependence of components that are not apparent under normal conditions [Chomsky, 1968; Cicchetti, 1996; Cicchetti & Sroufe, 1976].

The empirical study of 'experiments of nature', such as being brought up in a maltreating home, enable us to isolate components of the developmental system and clarify the structural organization of the normal system. The ecological conditions associated with child maltreatment represent a severe deviation from the average expectable environment [Cicchetti & Lynch, 1995]. Research on child maltreatment can inform, affirm, and challenge developmental theory through elucidating the conditions necessary for normal emotional development and healthy adaptation. In particular, the study of maltreated children affords researchers the opportunity to examine how atypical emotional experiences and early trauma affect the functioning of emotion systems.

A major advantage of studying emotional development in maltreated children is that whereas the basic emotional environment experienced by most typically developing nonmaltreated children may be so invariant that environmental/experiential influences are overlooked [Pollak, Cicchetti, Hornung & Reed, 2000], the emotional experiences of maltreated children enable researchers to parse the relative contributions of experience and learning versus innate internal predispositions. In comparison with nonmaltreating parents, maltreating parents exhibit less positive emotion and more negative emotion, including episodes of intense hostility and interpersonal threat [Cicchetti & Valentino, 2006; Pollak et al., 2000; Rogosch, Cicchetti, Shields & Toth, 1995]. Moreover, maltreating parents are more likely to isolate themselves and their families from others, thereby minimizing the number of nonparental models of emotional communication to whom their children are exposed [Pollak et al., 2000]. Since brain development occurs most rapidly during the first years of life [Stiles, 2008], these aberrant emotional experiences may eventuate in neuropathological connections that undermine effective emotion expression, emotion perception/recognition, emotion regulation, emotion processing, and emotion understanding in maltreated children [Cicchetti, 2002].

In this chapter, we review the literature on emotional development in maltreated children. Given the severe disturbances in the average expectable environment provided in maltreating families, considerable evidence has mounted to demonstrate the detrimental effects of maltreatment on children's emotional development. Specifically, as discussed below, maltreated children have shown deviations in a number of components of emotion systems. These include emotion expression [Gaensbauer, Mrazek & Harmon, 1981], emotion recognition [Camras, Sachs-Alter & Ribordy, 1996; Pollak et al., 2000], emotion regulation [Kim-Spoon, Cicchetti & Rogosch, 2013], emotion understanding [Shipman & Zeman, 1999; Shipman, Zeman, Penza & Champion, 2000] and emotion communication [Beeghly & Cicchetti, 1994]. In the penultimate section, we propose future research directions for research on emotional development in maltreated children. Finally, we discuss the implications that research on emotional development in maltreated children has for implementing and evaluating preventative interventions.

Emotion Expression

Divergence in maltreated children's emotional expression has been noted as early as 3 months of age, where severely physically abused infants have evinced increased rates of fearfulness, anger, and sadness during mother-infant interactions [Gaensbauer et al., 1981]. The expression of fear and anger is a particularly salient finding considering that the normative ontogenic development of these affects does not typically occur until approximately 7–9 months of age [Sroufe, 1996]. In contrast, neglected infants displayed an attenuated range of emotional expression and an increased duration of negative affect as compared to nonmaltreated infants [Gaensbauer et al., 1981].

To examine the affective input that maltreated children receive, Camras et al. [1988, 1990] investigated the facial expressions of maltreating and nonmaltreating mothers. When asked to deliberately pose discrete facial expressions, maltreating mothers' productions of emotion faces were less readily identified by observers than were the expressions of nonmaltreating mothers [Camras et al., 1988]. During mother-child interactions, maltreating mothers differed from nonmaltreating mothers with regard to the expression of sadness [Camras et al., 1990]. Taken together, the emotion displays of abused and neglected infants highlight the centrality of interactions with caregivers in shaping the development of affect expression or affect differentiation. Furthermore, maternal emotional expression ability contributes to their children's ability to recognize facial emotion [Camras et al., 1990]. Thus, within their first 3 months of life, maltreated children are already at risk for developing different emotion regulation trajectories.

Emotion Recognition

Accurate emotion recognition is critical because it represents the early use of social cues on which children's subsequent interpretations and behavioral responses will depend [Pollak et al., 2000]. The identification of the basic emotions from both facial and contextual cues is normatively mastered by the preschool years. Unfortunately, maltreated children evince lower accuracy in recognizing emotions than nonmaltreated children, even after controlling for receptive linguistic ability [Pollak et al., 2000].

Developmentally, early information processing limitations require children to focus their attention on the most salient aspects of their environment [Bjorklund, 1997]. For children who are physically abused, displays of anger may signal imminent threat. Consequently, Pollak et al. [2000] hypothesized that 3- to 5-year-old physically abused children would exhibit an increased sensitivity to anger-related cues perhaps also resulting in decreased attention to other types of emotional cues. Confirming their hypothesis, physically abused preschoolers perceived angry faces as more salient and distinctive relative to other emotions (e.g., sadness, fear, disgust, happiness) on a perceptual scaling task, whereas nonmaltreated comparison children did not show this pattern. Moreover, when physically abused children were instructed to match facial expressions to emotional situations, they demonstrated a lower threshold for detecting anger compared to demographically comparable nonmaltreated peers. Further studies have confirmed this heightened vigilance to anger in physically abused children: They display broader perceptual category boundaries for perceiving anger [Pollak & Kistler, 2002], they require less visual information to detect the presence of angry facial expressions [Pollak & Sinha, 2002], and they recognize anger earlier in the formation of the facial expression when fewer cues are available [Pollak, Messner, Kistler & Cohn, 2009] compared to nonmaltreated children.

Processing of Affective Facial Expressions

Neuroscientific and psychophysiological studies also provide evidence that physically abused children allocate more attentional resources to the detection of anger, but respond similarly to nonmaltreated children when attending to happy and fearful faces. Specifically, measurement of cognitive event-related brain potentials (ERPs) indicates that school-aged maltreated children display larger P3b amplitude when their attention is directed toward angry, as opposed to happy or fearful targets [Pollak, Cicchetti, Klorman & Brumaghim, 1997]. P3b amplitude varies as a function of task relevance and has been used to clarify specific cognitive operations such as the evaluation of stimulus significance [Johnson, 1993]. It also may be reflective of processes involved in the updating of mental representations in working memory. In general, such psychophysiological processes serve to maintain representations of one's environment by highlighting events that are significant. Moreover, this pattern of response appears to be specific to anger rather than to negative emotions, such as fear [Pollak, Klorman, Thatcher & Cicchetti, 2001]. Similarly, findings indicate that maltreated children exhibit brain-based abnormalities in the processing of facial affect as early as 15 to 30 to 42 months of age [Cicchetti & Curtis, 2005; Curtis & Cicchetti, 2011, 2013].

Thus, physically abused children do not have emotion recognition or affective information-processing deficits in a global sense; rather, differential processing of emotion appears to be specific to anger. It is certainly conceivable that an increased sensitivity to anger might be adaptive for physically abused children, as it would allow for hypervigilant detection of imminent harm, but successful regulation includes the capacity for flexibility and control over attention. The failure of regulatory capacities that enable flexibility and control make what is adaptive in the maltreating home maladaptive when generalized to more normative social contexts [Pollak, 2008].

Pollak and Tolley-Schell [2003] posited that early experiences of abuse may alter the development of perceptual systems by decreasing the minimum amount of threat-related stimulation needed to engage focused attention on the threat-inducing stimuli. If physically abused children respond more quickly and/or strongly to signals of threat, then problems disengaging attention away from anger may emerge. Using a selective attention paradigm with an affective component, both physiological and behavioral measures were employed to assess 8- to 11-year-old children's orienting reaction and response time during valid trials, and children's disengagement reaction and response time during invalid trials [Pollak & Tolley-Schell, 2003]. Psychophysiological data confirmed the hypothesis that physically abused children demonstrate a selective increase in ERP response (as measured by P3b) on invalid angry trials, providing evidence that increased attentional resources were required to disengage from previously cued angry faces only. Physically abused children also demonstrated faster reaction times in the valid angry condition, consistent with the notion that abused children orient rapidly to cues primed by anger. There were no differences, however, in physically abused children's psychophysiological responses or reaction times to happy trials, providing further support for a specific or differential deficit involving attentional processing of anger. Thus, the nature of the experiences that maltreated children encounter during their lives contribute to a particular class of emotional stimuli becoming more salient (anger cues); leading to quicker orienting and detection as well as greater difficulty in disengagement.

Conceivably, the early expression of fear, anger, and sadness that emerges within the first 3 months of life may reflect deviations at the neural level, whereby negative-affect processing synapses are strengthened, leading to later differences in attentional control in response to anger-related cues. These emotion recognition and processing biases which seem to have their roots in the first year of life, could render physically abused children vulnerable to unsuccessful resolution of stage-salient developmental tasks. For example, one possible pathway to maladaptation might include a predisposition for developing an atypical pattern of attachment, especially since the development of disorganized attachment has been linked to frightened or frightening parenting [Hesse & Main, 2006].

At subsequent developmental periods, physically abused children might manifest social information-processing deficits and difficulties with peer relationships. Social information-processing biases that are prevalent among abused children's peer relations indicate that maltreated children are more, rather than less, likely to respond to angry or aggressive emotional cues [Dodge, Pettit & Bates, 1997; Rieder & Cicchetti, 1989; Teisl & Cicchetti, 2008]. Such social information processing biases are consistent with the attentional biases exhibited by abused children in response to expressions of anger [Pollak & Tolley-Schell, 2003].

Behavioral and psychophysiological evidence of maltreated children's differential processing of affective information suggests that early experience influences subsequent emotional development and shapes implicated brain circuitry. The effects observed among maltreated children may reflect experience-dependent processes that involve the fine-tuning of attention, learning, perceptual, and memory systems that facilitate the rapid identification of anger [Pollak, 2008].

Emotion Regulation

Defined as the monitoring, evaluating, and modifying of emotional reactions for the purpose of achieving individual goals, emotion regulation optimizes one's adaptive engagement with the environment [Thompson, Lewis & Calkins, 2008]. Because the ability to autonomously regulate one's emotions is believed to emerge from early parent-child relations [Camras et al., this vol.; Lemerise et al., this vol.; Sroufe, 1996], maltreatment poses a serious risk to children's development of emotion regulation. In maltreating families, parents provide less support and scaffolding when their children are upset – limiting children's ability to learn constructive strategies to regulate their emotional states. Maltreating caregivers also engage their children less often in emotional discussions [Edwards, Shipman & Brown, 2005; Shipman & Zeman, 1999], demonstrate impaired capacity to understand their children's affective expression, and offer less anger management strategies relative to typical parents [Shipman & Zeman, 2001]. An unpredictable and disorganized environment, such as those found in maltreating homes [Howes, Cicchetti, Toth & Rogosch, 2000], would make children particularly vulnerable to frequent negative emotional experiences, including anger, frustration, reactivity, and irritability from caregivers. Accordingly, maltreated children are likely to experience overwhelming emotional arousal that leads to difficulties managing and processing negative emotions.

Maughan and Cicchetti [2002] applied a person-oriented approach to assess how different maltreatment experiences (i.e., physical abuse and neglect), in conjuction with a history of exposure to interadult violence, may exert an impact on 4- to 6-year-olds' ability to regulate their emotions in response to live simulations of interadult anger directed toward their mother. Results indicated that approximately 80% of the maltreated children evidenced dysregulated emotion patterns (i.e., undercontrolled/ambivalent or over-controlled/unresponsive), in comparison to only 36% of the nonmaltreated children [Maughan & Cicchetti, 2002]. The emotional response patterns of maltreated children provide support for Davies and Cummings' [1994] emotional security hypothesis proposing that a child's feelings of emotional security are largely determined by familial relations in the early caregiving environment. With regard to maltreated children, unpredictable and threatening interpersonal exchanges often characterize their early family environment, resulting in children's increased emotional insecurity. Without adequate emotional security, a child's self-regulatory abilities may be easily overwhelmed by environmental stressors, leading to the development of over- and underregulation, as exemplified by the high rate of emotional dysregulation patterns found among maltreated children.

Maladaptive emotion regulation also has been observed among maltreated children during peer interactions. Shields and Cicchetti [1998] demonstrated the relation of emotion dysregulation and attention to the development of reactive aggression among maltreated children. Specifically, during their interactions with peers, maltreated children exhibited higher rates of aggression, as well as increased distractibility, overactivity and poor concentration (characteristic of children with deficits in attention modulation). Furthermore, attention deficits mediated the effects of maltreatment on emotional lability/negativity, inappropriate affect, and attenuated emotion regulation. Therefore, it seems that attention processes (which may have their roots in early anger recognition biases that develop during infancy) may interact with negative representations and maladaptive social information processing to foster emotional negativity and reactivity among maltreated children. This in turn seems to provoke reactive aggression, particularly among children with histories of physical abuse.

Additional evidence suggests that emotional dysregulation may mediate the increased risk of bullying and victimization that has been noted among maltreated children [Shields & Cicchetti, 2001], highlighting how the internalization of salient aspects of the early caregiving relationship may have maladaptive implications among these children. As maltreated children are victimized by parents, they may develop a working model of relationships as dangerous and malevolent that incorporates the roles of both bully and victim. These cognitive-affective structures may then guide behaviors and peer interactions, promoting emotional construction of atypical emotional responsiveness and coloring children's interpretations of the behavior of social partners. Supporting this hypothesis, Shields, Ryan and Cicchetti [2001] found that 8- to 12-year-old maltreated children's representations of their caregivers were more negative/constricted and less positive/coherent than those of nonmaltreated children. Maladaptive caregiver representations were associated with greater emotion dysregulation, aggression, and peer rejection, whereas positive/coherent representations were related to prosocial behavior and peer preferences as indexed by peer ratings and adult observations.

Problems in regulating emotions have also been found to increase the likelihood of internalizing mental health difficulties in maltreated children. Specifically, Kim and Cicchetti [2010] demonstrated that children with early experiences of abuse and neglect were more likely to display poor emotion regulation. Consequently, the maltreated children with poor emotion regulation were less likely to be accepted by peers and were likely to exhibit higher internalizing symptomatology 1 year later, even after controlling for initial levels of internalizing symptomatology. Kim-Spoon, Cicchetti and Rogosch [2013] conducted a longitudinal study from age 7 to age 10 examining the contributions of emotion regulation and emotion lability/negativity to internalizing symptomatology in a sample of maltreated and nonmaltreated children. Significant longitudinal mediation effects of maltreatment suggested that early maltreatment was associated with higher emotion lability/negativity (age 7) that contributed to poor emotion regulation (age 8) which in turn was predictive of increases in internalizing symptomatology (from ages 8 to 9). These results further demonstrated the potentially important roles of emotion regulation in the development of internalizing symptomatology, especially for children with high emotion lability/negativity.

Research on the biological sequelae of child maltreatment has begun to shed light on the neurological underpinnings of emotion regulation in these children. A brain structure that has been accorded a great deal of attention in neuroimaging studies of child maltreatment is the prefrontal cortex [e.g., DeBellis et al., 2002]. This structure is of particular interest to developmentalists because it reaches full maturation later in ontogeny and, hence, may be especially vulnerable to the early stress of child maltreatment. Moreover, because the prefrontal cortex is involved in emotion regulatory processes and has connections to a number of additional regulatory brain regions (e.g., the amygdala), it will be important to undertake studies investigating neurobiological functioning in maltreated children and adolescents.

Emotion Understanding

Emotion understanding is characterized by the ability to comprehend the sources of emotions, and the appropriate affective responses to emotional experiences [Thompson & Lagattuta, 2006]. In the context of normal development, emotion understanding has been shown to develop differentially depending on the quality of parent-child relationships [Ontai & Thompson, 2002], maternal affective expressivity [Ontai & Thompson, 2002], and the nature of the child's peer relations [Brown & Dunn, 1996]. Although emotion understanding has been widely examined in normative development, this domain has been relatively uncharted in child maltreatment research [Thompson & Lagattuta, 2006].

In a study of mothers and their 5- to 12-year-old children, maternal support has been demonstrated to mediate the relation between child neglect and emotion understanding [Edwards et al., 2005]. Moreover, mothers' discussion of antecedents and consequences of affective states to their children has been shown to be related to children's emotion understanding performance [Shipman & Zeman, 1999]. More recently, Perlman, Kalish and Pollak [2008] discovered that 5- and 6-year-old maltreated children exhibited significant impairments in emotion understanding. The maltreated children were significantly more likely to erroneously perceive negative affect (e.g., anger and sadness) as plausible consequences of positive events, yet performed similarly to comparison children in judging positive events as causes of positive affect. These findings suggest that the inconsistent and aberrant emotional experiences during early maltreatment limit the acquisition of emotional knowledge and lead to modifications in the children's reasoning about affective communication, source, and outcome. These results suggest that prior observations of hypervigilance to threat-related stimuli [Rieder & Cicchetti, 1989; Rogosch, Cicchetti & Aber, 1995] and a superior recognition of anger in maltreated children do not necessarily reflect more sophisticated comprehension of anger. Maltreated children may be more reactive to angry states rather than understanding their sources or outcomes. Although vigilance to anger is adaptive in the maltreating environment, it is highly likely to be maladaptive if utilized in other contexts.

Future Research Directions

The confluence of the research investigations conducted to date cohere in their demonstration that the experience of child abuse and neglect is detrimental to the emotional development of maltreated children. Specifically, maltreated children exhibit deficits in emotion recognition, the neural processing of facial affect expressions, emotion regulation, and emotion understanding. We next proffer a number of suggested topics we believe should be addressed in future research in the area of emotional development of maltreated children.

(1) More work needs to be conducted on the development of emotional expression in maltreated children with considerations of the specific period when maltreatment experience occurred. Ideally, this work should be longitudinal to ascertain whether the facial expressions of maltreated infants and children progress through the same longitudinal sequence as that of nonmaltreated youngsters. Careful coding of videotaped facial affects would enable researchers to determine whether the morphology of their emotion expressions is similar or different from that of children who have not experienced maltreatment. Such extensive investigation would afford opportunities to elucidate how maltreatment experiences at selective developmental periods may elicit differential outcomes in emotion expressivity.

(2) Additional investigations of maltreating mothers' encoding and decoding of emotion expressions are warranted. Are maltreating mothers' emotion encoding abilities on par with those of nonmaltreating mothers? Do maltreating mothers accurately decode and interpret the facial and other emotion expressions of their children? In this vein, do maltreating mothers differ in their emotion recognition competency when evaluating their own versus other children? Likewise, how accurate are maltreated children in decoding their mother's versus other's affect? Where do problems lie in the development of emotion synchrony between maltreating mothers and their children? How might these difficulties in affect synchrony interfere with maltreating infants' and children's ability to 'make meaning' out of their interactions with their mothers [Tronick & Beeghly, 2011]?

(3) There is a paucity of research on emotion or internal state language in maltreated children and their parents. Extant research findings suggest that maltreated toddlers, along with their mother, have developed an interaction style in which language predominantly functions as a medium to accomplish tasks rather than as a vehicle for social or affective exchanges [Beeghly & Cicchetti, 1994]. In addition, maltreated toddlers have been found to produce less internal state language about emotions and physiological states and less language about 'the self' more generally [Beeghly & Cicchetti, 1994]. These findings suggest the possibility that behavior problems may emerge when children are not able or willing to express their feelings. Furthermore, maltreated children's deficits in the pragmatic use of language for social sharing may present further challenges in their ability to develop close relationships and feel a sense of belongingness in later peer group formations.

Longitudinal research on the development of emotion language in maltreated toddlers and preschoolers, in concert with concurrent examination of internal state language use in maltreating mothers, would be a valuable addition to the understanding of the relation between maternal and child communication in a socioemotional context [Ng & Cicchetti, in preparation].

The significant gap in emotion understanding research that exists in the maltreatment literature leaves many unanswered questions. For example, it is unknown whether physically abused children show greater understanding of angry emotional states, in parallel to their heightened attentional allocation to anger, or whether these children will show broad emotion understanding deficits, indicating that enhanced detection of anger is an emotional reaction rather than a full comprehension of the affective state. Likewise, it is not clear whether neglected children will exhibit generalized emotion understanding deficits across affects, mirroring their general emotion-perception deficits. Investigating emotion understanding in abused and neglected children will provide greater clarity regarding how particular maltreatment experiences may shape the processing of emotional states and the allocation of attentional resources to specific affects. Furthermore, deviations in emotion understanding may help to explain the increased emotion dysregulation, aggression, and affect negativity exhibited by maltreated children. Consequently, future research on emotion understanding in maltreated children holds great promise for elucidating the development of affective-perceptual and cognitive processes and dysregulatory behaviors in the face of early emotional trauma.

Empirical investigations of emotional development in maltreated children who are functioning resiliently despite experiencing significant adversity can help to parse out the factors and processes whereby the negative emotional effects of trauma may be diminished. For example, positive emotion regulatory abilities have been found to be predictive of resilient functioning in maltreated children [Cicchetti, 2013]. This association of positive emotion with resilience is consistent with the broader scientific literature on psychosocial contributors to resilient functioning. Likewise, Curtis and Cicchetti [2007] discovered that resilient maltreated children evinced more positive emotionality as measured by left asymmetrical electroencephalogram activity across parietal brain regions. Moreover, adult observational ratings of emotion regulation also made a unique contribution to resilience in these children.

Another multilevel investigation conducted by Cicchetti and Rogosch [2007] found that the personality constructs of moderate ego control and ego resiliency, along with assessments of adrenal steroid hormones (i.e., cortisol, dehydroepiandrosterone), independently contributed to resilience, and that these predictors functioned differentially for maltreated and nonmaltreated children. For example, lower morning cortisol predicted higher resilient functioning for nonmaltreated children, whereas high morning cortisol was associated with higher resilient functioning for physically abused children. Furthermore, maltreated children with high resilience showed an atypical rise in dehydroepiandrosterone from morning to afternoon. To fully comprehend emotional development, both high-risk and resilient individuals from both typical and aberrant emotion environments need to be studied longitudinally so that developmental trajectories under optimal, average, and challenging circumstances can be tracked. Moreover, investigating affective functioning in resilient maltreated children is another important avenue for comprehending developmental continuities and discontinuities in emotion understanding.

Many strides in our knowledge of emotion systems in maltreated children can be made by undertaking integrative multilevel studies that incorporate concepts and methods from an array of disciplines. Such work would entail conducting longitudinal investigations of the transactional relations between and among molecular, genetic, neural, endocrine, immune, and the emotional domains as a function of developmental processes and timing of maltreatment onset. Given that the development of psychopathology both originates from and manifests itself through a multitude of factors and processes, future research on emotional development in maltreated children must strive to address it in its full complexity. The development of emotion systems in maltreated children, from information recognition and processing to the development of emotional regulatory strategies, emotion communication, and emotion understanding, is inextricably interwoven with the individual dispositions and social experiences of abused and neglected children. Since the emotional network itself is a multilevel neurobiological structure, future empirical research on the emotional development of maltreated children should increasingly become multilevel and interdisciplinary in nature.

Implications for Intervention and Conclusions

It is imperative that the scientific investigations of emotional development and the emotion neural network in children who have experienced maltreatment inform prevention and intervention efforts. The translation of sound empirical research into early interventions may eradicate or diminish the adverse effects of child maltreatment and contribute to the development of new strategies for coping with emotional states and for reorganizing the emotion information network of abused and neglected children.

For example, children who have been maltreated exhibit brain-based abnormalities in processing facial affect. These findings underscore the importance of providing early preventive interventions to children who have experienced maltreatment in order to avert the potential cascade of effects this experience may have on brain development and functioning. Theoretically and developmentally informed early preventive interventions can serve to move young maltreated children onto more adaptive developmental pathways, thereby mitigating their risk for developing psychopathology [Cicchetti, Rogosch & Toth, 2006; Cicchetti, Rogosch, Toth & Stugle-Apple, 2011]. ERP studies of affect expression processing in maltreated children suggest that interventions might focus on training in facial affect recognition. Such emphasis on coaching maltreated children in the ability to vocally and facially express emotions appropriately would help improve socioemotional development. Although such training would likely be at a very basic level for infants and young children, later in development more intensive efforts might attempt to change the salience and/or representation of emotion – in particular, that of anger.

Interventions targeting parenting methods may be additional avenues to improve emotional development in maltreated children. For example, maltreating parents could also profit from interventions focusing on emotion coaching, emotion socialization, and emotion communication. These interventions facilitate sensitive parent-child relationships and may help to eliminate or reduce the deviations in maltreated children's emotional development. Moreover, attachment-informed interventions such as child-parent psychotherapy could focus on altering representations of cognitive and emotional processes [e.g., Toth, Maughan, Manly, Spagnola & Cicchetti, 2002]. In effect, parent-guided interventions could positively impact the socioemotional dynamics between the caregiver and their offspring, creating more social learning opportunities and emotional support for the child.

Additionally, it would be elucidating to include baseline and post-intervention measures of ERPs and/or of MRI/fMRI elicited by tasks that tap emotion systems in multilevel evaluations of intervention efficacy. Given that behavioral and representational changes have been shown to improve in attachment-informed interventions, it also would be important to ascertain if ERPs, a manifestation of brain functioning, or structural and functional neuroimaging parameters exhibit postintervention improvement.

Undeniably, there is a need for sufficient breadth in prevention and intervention programs to address the complex developmental consequences of maltreated children, as well as the parenting practices, relationship disturbances, and extensive physical and mental health needs of these families. Policy-relevant decisions concerning the design and implementation of evidenced-based interventions to address the socioemotional difficulties of maltreated children, as well as the formation of strategies to evaluate the efficacy of these intervention efforts, would profit immeasurably from continued methodologically rigorous, multilevel biological and psychological research on emotional development.

Acknowledgments

Work on this chapter was supported in part by grants from the National Institute of Mental Health (MH083979) and the Spunk Fund, Inc. to Dante Cicchetti.

References

Beeghly, M., & Cicchetti, D. (1994). Child maltreatment, attachment, and the self-system: Emergence of an internal state lexicon in toddlers at high social risk. *Development and Psychopathology, 6,* 5–30.

Bjorklund, D.F. (1997). The role of immaturity in human development. *Psychological Bulletin, 122,* 153–169.

Brown, J.R., & Dunn, J. (1996). Continuities in emotion understanding from 3–6 years. *Child Development, 67,* 789–802.

Camras, L.A., Ribordy, S., Hill, J., Martino, S., Sachs, V., Spaccarelli, S., & Stefani, R. (1990). Maternal facial behavior and the recognition and production of emotional expression by maltreated and non-maltreated children. *Developmental Psychology, 26,* 304–312.

Camras, L.A., Ribordy, S., Hill, J., Martino, S., Spaccarelli, S., & Stefani, R. (1988). Recognition and posing of emotional expressions by abused children and their mothers. *Developmental Psychology, 24,* 776–781.

Camras, L.A., Sachs-Alter, E., & Ribordy, S. (1996). Emotion understanding in maltreated children: Recognition of facial expressions and integration with other emotion cues. In M. Lewis & M.W. Sullivan (Eds.), *Emotional development in atypical children* (pp. 203–225). Hillsdale: Lawrence Erlbaum Associates.

Chomsky, N. (1968). *Language and mind.* New York: Harcourt Brace Jovanovich.

Cicchetti, D. (1984). The emergence of developmental psychopathology. *Child Development, 55,* 1–7.

Cicchetti, D. (1990). A historical perspective on the discipline of developmental psychopathology. In J. Rolf, A. Masten, D. Cicchetti, K. Nuechterlein & S. Weintraub (Eds.), *Risk and protective factors in the development of psychopathology* (pp. 2–28). New York: Cambridge University Press.

Cicchetti, D. (1993). Developmental psychopathology: Reactions, reflections, projections. *Developmental Review, 13,* 471–502.

Cicchetti, D. (1996). Child maltreatment: Implications for developmental theory. *Human Development, 39,* 18–39.

Cicchetti, D. (2002). The impact of social experience on neurobiological systems: Illustration from a constructivist view of child maltreatment. *Cognitive Development, 17,* 1407–1428.

Cicchetti, D. (2013). Resilient functioning in maltreated children: Past, present, and future perspectives. *Journal of Child Psychology and Psychiatry, 54,* 402–422.

Cicchetti, D., Ackerman, B., & Izard, C. (1995). Emotions and emotion regulation in developmental psychopathology. *Development and Psychopathology, 7,* 1–10.

Cicchetti, D., & Curtis, W.J. (2005). An event-related potential study of the processing of affective facial expressions in young children who experienced maltreatment during the first year of life. *Development and Psychopathology, 17,* 641–677.

Cicchetti, D., & Lynch, M. (1995). Failures in the expectable environment and their impact on individual development: The case of child maltreatment. In D. Cicchetti & D.J. Cohen (Eds.), *Developmental psychopathology: Risk, disorder, and adaptation* (pp. 32–71). New York: John Wiley & Sons, Inc.

Cicchetti, D., & Rogosch, F.A. (2007). Personality, adrenal steroid hormones, and resilience in maltreated children: A multilevel perspective. *Development and Psychopathology, 19,* 787–809.

Cicchetti, D., Rogosch, F.A., & Toth, S.L. (2006). Fostering secure attachment in infants in maltreating families through preventive interventions. *Development and Psychopathology, 18,* 623–650.

Cicchetti, D., Rogosch, F.A., Toth, S.L., & Sturge-Apple, M.L. (2011). Normalizing the development of cortisol regulation in maltreated infants through preventive interventions. *Development and Psychopathology, 23,* 789–800.

Cicchetti, D., & Schneider-Rosen, K. (1984). Theoretical and empirical considerations in the investigation of the relationship between affect and cognition in atypical populations of infants: Contributions to the formulation of an integrative theory of development. In C. Izard, J. Kagan & R. Zajonc (Eds.), *Emotions, cognition, and behavior* (pp. 366–406). New York: Cambridge University Press.

Cicchetti, D., & Sroufe, L.A. (1976). The relationship between affective and cognitive development in Down's syndrome infants. *Child Development, 47,* 920–929.

Cicchetti, D., & Valentino, K. (2006). An ecological transactional perspective on child maltreatment: Failure of the average expectable environment and its influence upon child development. In D. Cicchetti & D.J. Cohen (Eds.), *Developmental Psychopathology.* Vol. 3 (pp. 129–201). New York: Wiley.

Curtis, W.J., & Cicchetti, D. (2007). Emotion and resilience: A multilevel investigation of hemispheric electroencephalogram asymmetry and emotion regulation in maltreated and nonmaltreated children. *Development and Psychopathology, 19,* 811–840.

Curtis, W. J., & Cicchetti, D. (2011). Affective facial expression processing in young children who have experienced maltreatment during the first year of life: An event-related potential study. *Development and Psychopathology, 23,* 373–395.

Curtis, W.J., & Cicchetti, D. (2013). Affective facial expression processing in 15 month-old infants who have experienced maltreatment: An event-related study. *Child Maltreatment.* E-pub ahead of print.

Davies, P., & Cummings, E.M. (1994). Marital conflict and child adjustment: An emotional security hypothesis. *Psychological Bulletin, 116*, 387–411.
DeBellis, M.D., Keshavan, M.S., Shifflett, H., Iyengar, S., Beers, S.R., Hall, J., & Moritz, G. (2002). Brain structures in pediatric maltreatment-related posttraumatic stress disorder: A sociodemographically matched study. *Biological Psychiatry, 52*, 1066–1078.
Dodge, K., Pettit, G., & Bates, J.E. (1997). How the experience of early physical abuse leads children to become chronically aggressive. In D. Cicchetti & S.L. Toth (Eds.), *Rochester Symposium on Developmental Psychopathology*. Vol. 8 (pp. 263–288). Rochester: University of Rochester Press.
Edwards, A., Shipman, K., & Brown, A. (2005). The socialization of emotional understanding: A comparison of neglectful and nonneglectful mothers and their children. *Child Maltreatment, 10*, 293–304.
Gaensbauer, T., Mrazek, D., & Harmon, R. (1981). Emotional expression in abused and/or neglected infants. In N. Frude (Ed.), *Psychological approaches to child abuse* (pp. 120–135). Totowa: Rowman and Littlefield.
Hesse, P., & Cicchetti, D. (1982). Perspectives on an integrated theory of emotional development. *New Directions for Child Development, 16*, 3–48.
Hesse, E., & Main, M. (2006). Frightened, threatening, and dissociative parental behavior in low-risk samples: Description, discussion, and interpretations. *Development and Psychopathology, 18*, 309–343.
Howes, P.W., Cicchetti, D., Toth, S.L., & Rogosch, F.A. (2000). Affective, structural, and relational characteristics of maltreating families: A systems perspective. *Journal of Family Psychology, 14*, 95–110.
Johnson, R. (1993). On the neural generators of the P300 component of the event-related potential. *Psychophysiology, 30*, 90–97.
Kaplan, B. (1966). The study of language in psychiatry: The comparative developmental approach and its application to symbolization and language in psychopathology. In S. Arieti (Ed.), *American handbook of psychiatry* (pp. 659–688). New York: Basic Books.
Kim, J., & Cicchetti, D. (2010). Longitudinal pathways linking child maltreatment, emotion regulation, peer relations, and psychopathology. *Journal of Child Psychology and Psychiatry, 51*, 706–716.
Kim-Spoon, J., Cicchetti, D., & Rogosch, F.A. (2013). A longitudinal study of emotion regulation, emotion lability-negativity, and internalizing symptomatology in maltreated and nonmaltreated children. *Child Development, 84*, 512–527.
Maughan, A., & Cicchetti, D. (2002). The impact of child maltreatment and interadult violence on children's emotion regulation abilities. *Child Development, 73*, 1525–1542.
Ng, R., & Cicchetti, D. (in preparation). The development of internal state language in maltreating and non-maltreating mothers offspring.
Ontai, L.L., & Thompson, R.A. (2002). Patterns of attachment and maternal discourse effects on children's emotion understanding from 3 to 5 years of age. *Social Development, 11*, 433–450.
Perlman, S.B., Kalish, C.W., & Pollak, S.D. (2008). The role of maltreatment experience in children's understanding of the antecedents of emotion. *Cognition and Emotion, 22*, 651–670.
Pollak, S.D. (2008). Mechanisms linking early experience and the emergence of emotions: Illustrations from the study of maltreated children. *Current Directions in Psychological Science, 17*, 370–375.
Pollak, S.D., Cicchetti, D., Hornung, K., & Reed, A. (2000). Recognizing emotion in faces: Developmental effects of child abuse and neglect. *Developmental Psychology, 36*, 679–688.
Pollak, S.D., Cicchetti, D., Klorman, R., & Brumaghim, J. (1997). Cognitive brain event-related potentials and emotion processing in maltreated children. *Child Development, 68*, 773–787.
Pollak, S.D., & Kistler, D.J. (2002). Early experience is associated with the development of categorical representations for facial expressions of emotion. *Proceedings of the National Academy of Sciences, 99*, 9072–9076.
Pollak, S.D., Klorman, R., Thatcher, J.E., & Cicchetti, D. (2001). P3b reflects maltreated children's reactions to facial displays of emotion. *Psychophysiology, 38*, 267–274.
Pollak, S.D., Messner, M., Kistler, D.J., & Cohn, J.F. (2009). Development of perceptual expertise in emotion recognition. *Cognition, 110*, 242–247.
Pollak, S.D., & Sinha, P. (2002). Effects of early experience on children's recognition of facial displays of emotion. *Developmental Psychology, 38*, 784–791.
Pollak, S.D., & Tolley-Schell, S.A. (2003). Selective attention to facial emotion in physically abused children. *Journal of Abnormal Psychology, 112*, 323–338.
Rieder, C., & Cicchetti, D. (1989). Organizational perspective on cognitive control functioning and cognitive-affective balance in maltreated children. *Developmental Psychology, 25*, 382–393.
Rogosch, F.A., Cicchetti, D., & Aber, J.L. (1995). The role of child maltreatment in early deviations in cognitive and affective processing abilities and later peer relationship problems. *Development and Psychopathology, 7*, 591–609.
Rogosch, F.A., Cicchetti, D., Shields, A., & Toth, S.L. (1995). Parenting dysfunction in child maltreatment. In M.H. Bornstein (Ed.), *Handbook of parenting, Vol. 4: Applied and practical parenting* (pp. 127–159). Hillsdale: Lawrence Erlbaum Associates, Inc.
Rutter, M. (1986). Child psychiatry: Looking 30 years ahead. *Journal of Child Psychology and Psychiatry, 27*, 803–840.
Shields, A., & Cicchetti, D. (1998). Reactive aggression among maltreated children: The contributions of attention and emotion dysregulation. *Journal of Clinical Child Psychology, 27*, 381–395.
Shields, A., & Cicchetti, D. (2001). Parental maltreatment and emotion dysregulation as risk factors for bullying and victimization in middle childhood. *Journal of Clinical Child Psychology, 30*, 349–363.
Shields, A., Ryan, R.M., & Cicchetti, D. (2001). Narrative representations of caregivers and emotion dysregulation as predictors of maltreated children's rejection by peers. *Developmental Psychology, 37*, 321–337.
Shipman, K.L., & Zeman, J. (1999). Emotional understanding: A comparison of physically maltreating and nonmaltreating mother-child dyads. *Journal of Clinical Child Psychology, 28*, 407–417.
Shipman, K.L., & Zeman, J. (2001). Socialization of children's emotion regulation in mother-child dyads: A developmental psychopathology perspective. *Development and Psychopathology, 13*, 317–336.

Shipman, K.L., Zeman, J., Penza, S., & Champion, K. (2000). Emotion management skills in sexually maltreated and nonmaltreated girls: A developmental psychopathology perspective. *Development and Psychopathology, 12*, 47–62.

Sroufe, L.A. (1990). Considering normal and abnormal together: The essence of developmental psychopathology. *Development and Psychopathology, 2*, 335–347.

Sroufe, L.A. (1996). Emotional development: The organization of emotional life in the early years. New York: Cambridge University Press.

Stiles, J. (2008). The fundamentals of brain development: Integrating nature and nurture. Cambridge: Harvard University Press.

Teisl, M., & Cicchetti, D. (2008). Physical abuse, cognitive and emotional processes, and aggressive/disruptive behavior problems. *Social Development, 16*, 1–23.

Thompson, R., & Lagattuta, K.H. (2006). Feeling and understanding: Early emotional development. In K. McCartney & D. Phillips (Eds.), *Blackwell Handbook of Early Childhood Development* (pp. 317–338). Malden: Blackwell Publishing.

Thompson, R.A., Lewis, M.D., & Calkins, S.D. (2008). Reassessing emotion regulation. *Child Development Perspectives, 2*, 124–131.

Toth, S.L., Maughan, A., Manly, J.T., Spagnola, M., & Cicchetti, D. (2002). The relative efficacy of two interventions in altering maltreated preschool children's representational models: Implications for attachment theory. *Development and Psychopathology, 14*, 777–808.

Tronick, E., & Beeghly, M. (2011). Infants' meaning-making and the development of mental health problems. *American Psychologist, 66*, 107–119.

Dante Cicchetti, PhD
Institute of Child Development, University of Minnesota
51 E. River Rd.
Minneapolis, MN 55455 (USA)
E-Mail cicchett@umn.edu

Hansen Lagattuta K (ed): Children and Emotion. New Insights into Developmental Affective Sciences.
Contrib Hum Dev. Basel, Karger, 2014, vol 26, pp 42–56 (DOI: 10.1159/000354350)

Temperament and Attention as Core Mechanisms in the Early Emergence of Anxiety

Koraly Pérez-Edgar · Bradley Taber-Thomas · Eran Auday · Santiago Morales

The Pennsylvania State University, University Park, Pa., USA

Abstract

Anxiety is a pervasive, impairing, and early appearing form of psychopathology. Even when anxiety remits, children remain at a two- to threefold increased risk for the later emergence of a mood disorder. Therefore, it is imperative to identify and examine underlying mechanisms that may shape early emerging patterns of behavior that are associated with anxiety. One of the strongest and first visible risk factors is childhood temperament. In particular, children who are behaviorally inhibited or temperamentally shy are more likely to exhibit signs of anxiety by adolescence. However, not all shy children do so, despite the early risk. We know that attention mechanisms, particularly the presence of attention biases toward or away from threat, can play a critical role in the emergence of anxiety. The current chapter will bring together these separate lines of research to examine the ways in which attention can modulate the documented link between early temperament and later anxiety. In doing so, the chapter will highlight multiple levels of analysis that focus on the behavioral, cognitive, and neural mechanisms in the temperament-attention-anxiety network. The chapter will help identify both markers and mechanisms of risk, supporting future work aimed at improving theory and intervention by focusing on attention biases to environmental threat.

Children can differ fundamentally in the ways in which they view and approach the world around them. While some children eagerly embrace the ambiguities and uncertainties of their environments as opportunities for discovery and surprise, other children retreat from the world, fleeing from these same uncertainties as markers of threat and risk. These patterns of behavior emerge from a complex equation incorporating in-born or biologically based emotional biases as well as learning processes deriving information from the environment. On the biological side of the equation, temperament-based patterns of approach and withdrawal have been linked to long-standing and stable profiles of socioemotional behavior [Fox, Henderson, Pérez-Edgar & White, 2008]. From an environmental perspective, we know that rearing environments, whether harsh and punitive or sensitive and nurturing, can also shape the ways in which children navigate their world [LoBue, 2013]. Adding to this complexity, the child's own world view – as seen in patterns of attentional and interpretive biases – can step in to modify how he or she responds to surrounding events [White, Helfinstein & Fox, 2010].

Given the complex systems simultaneously at work shaping individual trajectories of development it is not surprising that there are a multitude of developmental pathways that emerge from seemingly equivalent starting points. For example, although infant temperament is one of the strongest early predictors of anxiety [Fox & Pine, 2012; Pérez-Edgar & Fox, 2005], the majority of temperamentally shy children do not go on to manifest an anxiety disorder [Degnan & Fox, 2007]. This pattern of early risk leading to relative normalcy may act as the developmental equivalent of the statistical construct of regression to the mean. Over the course of time, development appears to smooth away the jagged edges of early risk through naturally occurring maturational, experiential, and social processes [Degnan, Almas & Fox, 2010].

For a subset of children, however, the risks evident early in life persist, calcifying into a pattern of maladaptation throughout childhood and into adulthood. Children appear to be more open to prevention and intervention [Pine, Helfinstein, Bar-Haim, Nelson & Fox, 2009]. As a result, it becomes increasingly difficult over time to redirect maladaptive trajectories. Thus, it is exceedingly important to identify and target the mechanisms at play early in life. These mechanisms – developmental tethers – bind children to specific trajectories and resist the normal ameliorative or 'smoothing away' process. From our lab's perspective, developmental tethers grow out the child's individual early traits or biases. These biases provoke an environmental response. The child processes and interprets these responses and frames subsequent behaviors based on the conclusions drawn. This pattern of provocation and response can become cyclical, growing progressively more entrenched (and biased) with each successive iteration.

The current chapter will bring together separate lines of research in temperament and attention to examine the ways in which attention can modulate the documented link between early temperament and later anxiety. In doing so, the chapter will highlight multiple levels of analysis that focus on the behavioral, cognitive, and neural mechanisms in the temperament-attention-anxiety network. This includes observed social behavior, clinical assessments, computer-based attention tasks, psychophysiological techniques, and neuroimaging. The chapter will help identify the markers and mechanisms of risk, supporting future work aimed at improving both theory and intervention.

Temperament and the Emergence of Anxiety

The psychological construct of temperament captures distinct patterns of neurochemistry, neuroanatomy, and gene expression which bias the ways in which individual children select, process, and respond to salient stimuli within their environments [Kagan, 2012; Rothbart, 2012]. Temperament-based differences are evident in the first months of life and may serve as the biological 'seed' for later personality [Rothbart, Ahadi & Evans, 2000]. Temperament-linked differences in outlook and behavior may also prove to be an important core mechanism for the later emergence of psychopathology [see also Hastings et al., this vol.]. In our laboratory, the focus has been on a specific temperamental type – behavioral inhibition. As infants, behaviorally inhibited children display signs of fear and wariness in response to unfamiliar stimuli [Schmidt et al., 1997] and this trait is marked by heightened vigilance, motor quieting, and withdrawal from novelty [Garcia Coll, Kagan & Reznick, 1984; Kagan, Reznick & Snidman, 1987]. By elementary school, many behaviorally inhibited children fear social circumstances, displaying poorly regulated social behavior and social reticence [Coplan, Rubin, Fox, Calkins & Stewart, 1994; Fox et al., 1995]. This, in turn, increases the likelihood of peer rejection, low self-esteem, and poor social competence [Rubin, Chen & Hymel, 1993; Schmidt, Fox, Schulkin & Gold, 1999]. Longitudinal studies of behavioral inhibition, and the broader construct of temperamental shyness, have found a marked increased risk for anxiety, particularly social anxiety, by mid-adolescence [Chronis-Tuscano et al., 2009; Kagan, Snidman, McManis & Woodward, 2001].

Despite this two- to threefold increase in risk for anxiety disorders, the majority of behaviorally inhibited children are not clinically anxious [Degnan & Fox, 2007]. Clearly, there must be a number of moderating influences that shape the trajectory from temperament to disorder. Past work suggests that parenting styles [Williams et al., 2009], parental anxiety levels [Biederman et al., 2001], and early schooling environment [Almas et al., 2011] all play a role in exacerbating or ameliorating early risk. Recently, a great deal of attention (pun intended) has focused on the role that systematic biases in early information processing patterns may play in shaping the emergence and course of anxiety. This will be the focus of the current chapter.

Attention, Attention Biases, and Socioemotional Development

Cognitive models of anxiety suggest that attention biases toward threat may be causally implicated in the development of anxiety disorders [MacLeod & Mathews, 2012]. Early attention can be thought of as a gatekeeper, controlling which aspects of the environment are taken in for further processing while filtering out of awareness irrelevant information. Thus, attention mechanisms are central to our ability to carry out adaptive goal-directed behaviors [Crick & Dodge, 1994]. However, attention, as the gate-keeper to downstream information processing mechanisms, must also possess the flexibility to redirect resources to unexpected or ambiguous events in the environment, particularly if they are potentially threatening in nature.

LoBue [2013] suggests that humans have perceptual biases for threatening stimuli that are evident in infancy and that may set the stage for learning – drawing attention to important stimuli in the environment. Importantly, these biases precede the development of fear for these potential threats [Oldfield, 1971] and seem to be independent of exposure to the threat in the child's environment [Penkunas & Coss, 2013]. While a perceptual sensitivity to threat may be a normative, evolutionary-based safety mechanism, there is growing evidence that a pronounced bias in this attention mechanism may lay the foundation for anxiety. Indeed, Todd et al. [2012] have argued that the predisposition to attend to specific emotion categories of the environment, 'affect-biased attention,' may act to shape broad patterns of socioemotional functioning by creating a habitual filtering process that privileges certain classes of information over other, less salient, classes.

Thus, hard-wired biases toward threat may, in some vulnerable populations, set the stage for later socioemotional difficulties. Indeed, many in the clinical literature make the clear declaration that attention plays a causal role in the emergence of anxiety and should therefore be a primary target of clinical intervention [Amir, Beard, Burns & Bomyea, 2009]. However, a number of important and critical open questions remain to be answered. For example, although general reviews and meta-analyses [Bar-Haim, Lamy, Pergamin, Bakermans-Kranenburg & van IJzendoorn, 2007] suggest a general pattern of attention bias *toward* threat, biases *away* from threat can emerge with manipulations of task parameters [Mogg, Bradley, De Bono & Painter, 1997; Mogg, Bradley, Miles & Dixon, 2004], specific diagnosis [Waters, Bradley & Mogg, in press], and exposure to stress prior to testing [Helfinstein, White, Bar-Haim &

Fox, 2008]. Thus, any clinical utility may be limited until we better understand the parameters that shape the strength and directionality of any underlying bias to threat. In addition, questions regarding the early emergence of attention biases (as discussed below) will need to be addressed in order to better understand the mechanisms underlying any observed patterns of bias.

Assessing Attention Biases to Threat

According to Wells and Matthews' [1996] Self-Regulatory Executive Function model of emotional disorder, attentional processes are involved in the maintenance of emotional disorder because attention biases 'diminish individuals' ability to process information that is incompatible with their fears' [Lonigan & Vasey, 2009]. Thus, a bias or vulnerability to threat may reduce one's capacity to integrate information that would diminish fear, engendering a cycle of negative information processing that maintains anxiety. Individuals who are able to break this cycle by overriding the draw of negative information (and preventing biased attention and hypervigilance) are less likely to exhibit anxiety [Mathews & MacLeod, 1994]. For example, attention bias towards threat may predict self-reported anxiety only for children with low ability to control attention who also have low levels of attentional or effortful control [Lonigan & Vasey, 2009; Susa, Pitică, Benga & Miclea, 2012].

Most investigations and clinical manipulations of attention bias use a variant of the dot-probe task, originally developed by MacLeod et al. [1986]. In this task, participants see two stimuli (one threatening and one nonthreatening) side-by-side, typically for 500 ms. The pair of stimuli is followed by a probe in one of the two stimulus locations. The participant is then required to respond as quickly and accurately as possible to the probe. Individuals display an attentional bias towards threat when they are faster to respond to the probes that replace the threatening stimuli compared to the probes that replace the non-threatening stimuli. This task has been modified on several occasions, changing the presentation time of the emotional stimuli, the position of the stimuli on screen (vertical vs. horizontal), and the stimuli itself. For example, the original task used threat-related and neutral words [MacLeod et al., 1986]. Most of the current literature, however, uses threat-related pictures, particularly facial expressions, as their emotional stimuli. An important limitation of the dot-probe task is its inability to determine if the attention bias is generated by a bias in initial orienting or difficulty disengaging from the threatening stimuli as the strength and directionality in bias is measured by a comparison of behavioral reaction times.

Nevertheless, in a meta-analysis, Bar-Haim et al. [2007] demonstrated that regardless of the discussed variations in the dot-probe task, and even when using other tasks (i.e. the Stroop and Posner tasks), anxious individuals show higher attentional bias towards threat-related stimuli compared with nonanxious individuals. In addition, evidence for the causal role of attention bias to threat and anxiety comes from experimental paradigms in which the attentional bias is modified towards or away from threat, showing changes in reported levels of anxiety and anxiety displays in laboratory observations [Bar-Haim, 2010; Hakamata et al., 2010]. Emerging data suggest that healthy and clinically anxious children also show changes in stress reactivity and anxiety when exposed to experimental manipulation of attention bias [Eldar et al., 2012; Eldar, Ricon & Bar-Haim, 2008].

Attention Biases, Behavioral Inhibition and Anxiety

The evidence reviewed above supports the relation between attentional biases and anxiety. However it does not address how these biases develop, the nature of the relation between these biases and anxiety symptoms, or if these biases are a precursor or a symptom of anxiety. To answer these questions, longitudinal studies assessing bias in attention over time and their relation across development to anxiety are required [Penkunas & Coss, 2013]. To our knowledge, these studies have yet to be published.

One way to begin answering such questions is to look at the relation of attention biases to threat at an early stage (i.e., children) and in populations at risk for anxiety (i.e., behavioral inhibition). Far fewer studies have examined differences in attentional bias and anxiety disorders in children compared to adults. However, the available evidence supports a similar pattern to the one observed in adults. Children and adolescents (ages 7–18) diagnosed with an anxiety disorder (generalized anxiety (GAD), social phobia, or separation anxiety) by clinical interview exhibited greater threat bias on the dot probe task using face stimuli relative to nonanxious comparisons [Roy et al., 2008]. Among children ages 8–12 clinically diagnosed as anxious (GAD, social phobia, separation anxiety, or specific phobia) those with higher levels of anxiety as assessed by self-report questionnaire exhibited threat bias on the faces dot probe [Waters, Henry, Mogg, Bradley & Pine, 2010]. Finally, among children with GAD, the magnitude of threat bias on the faces dot probe has been positively correlated with the levels of anxiety symptoms [Waters, Mogg, Bradley & Pine, 2008].

Studies examining the relation between attentional bias and populations at risk for anxiety such as behavioral inhibition are also scarce. Nevertheless, results in the expected direction have been found; adolescents (mean age 15 years) characterized by laboratory observations and maternal reports as high in behavioral inhibition as toddlers (14 and 24 months) and early in childhood (4 and 7 years) displayed higher attention bias to threat (angry faces) on the dot probe task compared to adolescents low in behavioral inhibition [Pérez-Edgar, Bar-Haim et al., 2010]. In addition, attention bias to threat moderated the relation between behavioral inhibition and withdrawn behaviors in adolescence as assessed by parent report, such that the relation between early behavioral inhibition and later social withdrawal was only evident in adolescents with an attention bias to threat. This relation between early inhibition and later withdrawal may emerge quite early as attention bias patterns moderate this link at age 5 [Pérez-Edgar et al., 2011].

The impact of attention on patterns of social behavior may be felt even earlier in development. In our earliest examination of attention as a developmental tether, Pérez-Edgar et al. [2010] evaluated patterns of sustained attention (related to vigilance) in 9-month-olds. Infants watched fixation video clips as a distractor stimulus was presented intermittently in the periphery of the visual field. Vigilance was assessed by subtracting the time spent attending to the distractor from the time spent sustaining attention on the fixation. This study found that the group of infants who exhibited greater vigilance (less sustained attention) was more likely to show increases in behavioral inhibition from 14 months to 7 years. Moreover, initial behavioral inhibition levels predicted social difficulties assessed during an observed social dyad interaction with an unfamiliar peer in adolescence only for the group displaying high levels of vigilance.

These findings illustrate that attentional biases are related to socioemotional functioning in a similar manner in adults, in pediatric anxiety, and in individuals simply at risk for the development for anxiety. Most importantly, these findings shed light on the possible role of attention bias in the etiology of anxiety disorders. Nevertheless, this area of research is in its earliest stages and much more needs to be explored. Questions remain regarding what aspects of attention are involved in the observed bias (e.g., orienting or disengagement) and how biases change across development in order to determine possible sensitive periods for the development of these biases and their influences on anxiety. In addition, we are only now beginning to understand the biological conduits that may shape observed biases and reflect their effect on behavior across development. While there are early signs of a genetic component linked to variations in serotonin [Beevers, Gibb, McGeary & Miller, 2007; Fox, Ridgewell & Ashwin, 2009; Gibb, Benas, Grassia & McGeary, 2009; Pérez-Edgar, Bar-Haim, McDermott, Gorodetsky, et al., 2010], our focus here will be on the known neural correlates of attention bias.

Neural and Psychophysiological Correlates of Attention Bias

In a pioneering examination of the biological correlates of attention bias to threat, Monk et al. [2006] investigated differences in brain activation between children and adolescents with GAD and healthy controls while completing the standard dot probe paradigm in the fMRI environment. The initial focus was on the limbic system, given the role of the amygdala in the circuitry of fear. Surprisingly, there were no differences in amygdala activity between groups. However, the GAD group, compared to the control group, showed higher levels of ventrolateral prefrontal cortex (vlPFC) activity to trials that contained an angry face. In addition, vlPFC was negatively associated with anxiety symptoms. Since the vlPFC has been widely involved in regulatory processes, these results suggest a compensatory executive response from the GAD group in order to regulate other regions such as amygdala, which may be overactive. No significant differences in activation were found between the two groups in response to either happy or neutral faces relative to baseline, arguing for possible specificity in the response to angry faces.

A follow-up study by the same group [Monk et al., 2008] found support for this conclusion by presenting GAD adolescents with masked (17 ms presentation) emotional stimuli. Here, GAD youth, compared to the control group, showed greater right amygdala activity and a strong negative coupling between amygdala and vlPFC during exposure to masked angry faces. In addition, this amygdala activity was correlated with anxiety symptoms, linking both reactive and regulatory processes with the emergence of anxiety. Again, no group differences were found for masked happy faces. Indeed, trait anxiety has been positively associated with attention bias towards threat and activation in the vlPFC during the dot-probe task [Telzer et al., 2008], perhaps reflecting the use of cognitive control to disengage from threatening stimuli. Recent work in young adults with a history of behavioral inhibition [Hardee et al., 2013] contributes to the emerging picture of strong connections between regulatory and reactive responses to threat, manifest in the PFC and the limbic system. This study found stronger connections between the vlPFC and limbic sites for the participants with a history of behavioral inhibition, relative to non-inhibited peers. In addition, the level of connectivity was associated with concurrent levels of internalizing symptoms only in young adults with a history of behavioral inhibition.

Importantly, a recent study has indicated that activation patterns within the vlPFC and amygdala subserving threat bias on the dot-probe task are stable across time [Britton et al., 2013]. This study presented participants, ages 8–17 years, with the dot-probe task in an fMRI scanner on two separate occasions (an average of approximately 4 months apart), and found that activation was strongly correlated across the two time points in the vlPFC and amygdala, but few other brain regions. This finding provides support for the proposition that attention biases to threat are linked to stable patterns of neural functioning. The data also suggest that any direct manipulations of attention bias (discussed in detail below) may be tracked by changes at the neural level.

While fMRI may help us localize the regions at play in attention biases to threat, the technology cannot help us with the chronometry – how biases in processing unfurl over time. In an attempt to examine the timing of attention biases, Eldar et al. [2010] examined differences in event-related potential (ERP) components between anxious and non-anxious young adults during the dot-probe task. This study found differences during the presentation of the emotional stimuli in components C1 and P2, suggesting that processing differences emerge within the first 100 ms of the task and implicating early, automatic attention biases. This pattern is in line with the fundamental role of affect-biased attention in processing, as Todd et al. [2012] suggested. More recently, Shechner et al. [2013] measured attention bias in anxious and nonanxious youth during a 10-second exposure to angry, happy, and neutral faces, using eye-tracking methodology to record eye movements. They found that anxious youth displayed greater attention bias to threat. In addition, this bias occurred in the earliest phases of stimulus presentation, as the anxious youth made more initial and faster fixations to angry faces than neutral faces.

Although our understanding of the psychological and biological mechanisms of attention bias to threat is relatively shallow, a newly thriving line of research is rapidly building on the available data [Britton et al., 2012; Hardee et al., 2013; Telzer et al., 2008]. Ongoing work [O'Toole & Dennis, 2013; Pérez-Edgar, Taber-Thomas, Thai, Morales & Danilo, 2013] is now beginning to examine the neural and psychophysiological correlates of attention bias before and after experimental intervention. These data will help us better understand the intriguing attention bias-anxiety relations first reported in the adult clinical literature.

Attention Bias in the Maintenance and Development of Anxiety

Given the relationship between biases in attention and anxiety [Bar-Haim et al., 2007] as well as temperamental risk for anxiety [Pérez-Edgar, Bar-Haim et al., 2010; Pérez-Edgar & Fox, 2005; Pérez-Edgar et al., 2011], it has been argued that attention biases to threat may play a causal role (a) during development in the pathophysiology of the disorder [Bar-Haim, 2010], and (b) in the ongoing maintenance of the disorder [MacLeod et al., 1986]. One possibility is that over time a bias in information attended to – for example, the selective favoring of negative information – alters affective information processing, which when compounded over time, results in affective disorder. This suggests that attention may be a fruitful target for preventive and therapeutic intervention for anxiety. In this vein, attention bias modification (ABM) training has been developed as a novel treatment that attempts to alter biases in attention and reduce the processing of negative information in the hopes of ameliorating or preventing internalizing problems [for reviews, see Bar-Haim, 2010; Hakamata et al., 2010].

Cognitive bias modification has been an important approach for alleviating and reducing vulnerability to anxiety [for review, see Britton et al., 2013]. Attention bias to threat presents an interesting target for treatment given the causal role it seems to play in internalizing problems. The reasoning behind such a treatment is that if attention bias to threat causes anxiety, training attention away from threat may ameliorate and reduce the risk of anxiety (fig. 1) [Fox & Pine, 2012; Mathews & MacLeod, 2002]. Although the published number of studies is small, Hakamata et al. [2010] conducted a meta-analysis looking at the impact of ABM on anxiety using 12 published ABM randomized controlled trials and found that ABM significantly reduces anxiety relative to a control task.

MacLeod et al. [2002] made an early attempt to assess the impact of modifying attention bias on anxiety. The authors reported two separate studies, both of 64 undergraduate participants who completed a dot-probe ABM or control task. Similar to the original dot-probe task [MacLeod et al., 1986], the repeated trials of the attention training task present two stimuli differing in va-

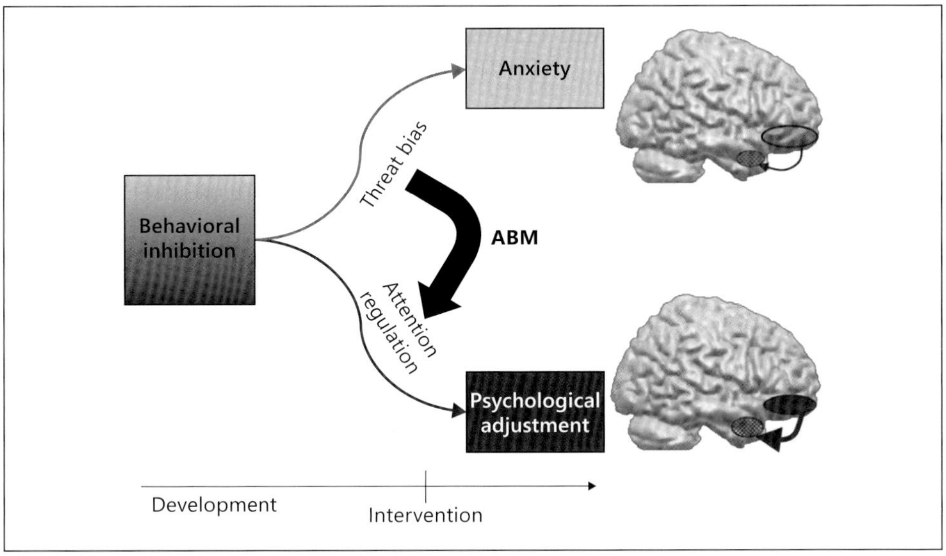

Fig. 1. Schematic representation of the relation between early risk, patterns of attention bias, and socioemotional outcomes. The developmental trajectory flows from left to right. Red denotes factors associated with anxiety and internalizing problems; blue denotes factors associated with psychological adjustment. Behavioral inhibition (left box, red and blue) is a temperamental risk factor for anxiety, but children with behavioral inhibition may or may not go on to develop anxiety. Attention bias toward threat acts as a tether pulling development toward anxiety and internalizing problems. Preventive intervention with ABM may enhance attention regulation, dislodging the developmental trajectory from the tether of threat bias and promoting psychological adjustment. The neural system underlying this process is indicated at the right; the ventrolateral prefrontal cortex (blue) exerts executive control over amygdala functioning, a process weakened in anxiety. Strengthening of this regulatory system may be the neural mechanism through which ABM exerts its effects on threat bias.

lence (negative/positive) followed immediately by a probe; the crucial difference is that in ABM the probe always (or usually) appears behind one of the stimulus types, thereby training attention toward that stimulus type. To demonstrate the viability of this paradigm, MacLeod et al. [2002] presented half of their participants with training away from threat and half with training toward threat. Results showed that attention training influenced attention biases as predicted, with the away group showing a bias away from threat, and the toward group showing a bias toward threat. Moreover, although state emotions were not immediately different between the groups, the 'away from threat' group showed significantly reduced negative emotional states than the 'toward threat group' when later exposed to a puzzle completion laboratory stressor paradigm. This exciting finding that training attention away from threat can reduce anxiety ignited interest in ABM as a potentially cost-effective, easy-to-administer, non-pharmacological tool for addressing anxiety.

Several studies have followed-up on these initial results, further demonstrating the impact of ABM on internalizing problems in different populations and with varying outcome measures. Much as with initial attention bias studies, ABM studies have also employed a variety of stimuli, including affective words, IAPS pictures, and standard emotion-face stimuli such as the NimStim set [Tottenham et al., 2009]. Currently, the majority of ABM studies employ faces as they are considered ecologically valid and can be used across the lifespan [Fox & Pine, 2012].

One study tested 94 socially anxious undergraduates, who performed a single session of dot-probe ABM with face (neutral/disgust) stimulus pairs with training toward the negative stimulus, or a control dot-probe task in which the probe was equally likely to appear behind one or the other stimulus type [Amir, Bomyea & Beard, 2010]. They found that the ABM group exhibited less attention bias to threat after training than the control group. Amir et al. [2010] then put all participants through a standard stress induction public-speaking challenge. As expected, the ABM group performed significantly better in the speech, which the authors interpreted as suggesting that the ABM group had lower levels of anxiety during this behavioral performance. In young adults with GAD (n = 29), Amir et al. [2009] found that an eight-session dot-probe ABM training (with text stimuli) reduced attention bias to threat and decreased anxiety on self-report and interviewer measures for participants trained away from threat (relative to those who performed the control task).

The evidence suggests that ABM can effectively impact internalizing symptoms. The questions of how clinically significant the impact of ABM is, and whether it lasts beyond the immediate window of the training, were addressed in a study by Schmidt et al. [2009]. The authors administered 8 sessions of ABM training (with face stimuli; neutral/disgust) or a control task to 36 patients with generalized social anxiety disorder, and found that 72% of patients in the ABM group versus 11% of control patients did not meet diagnostic criteria symptoms after training and the overall results were maintained at the 4-month follow-up. Thus, not only does ABM training have clinically significant effects on anxiety, but these effects also last at least on the order of months.

There is also evidence that computer-based ABM training has impacts on anxiety experience in real-world situations [See, MacLeod & Bridle, 2009]. In this clever study, 40 recent high school graduates were administered 15 daily sessions of internet-based word ABM or control task during the month prior to a stressful life event (travelling abroad to begin college). Both the ABM and control group exhibited increased state anxiety from pre-training to post-stressful event; however, relative to the control group, the ABM group exhibited a significantly smaller increase. That is, the impact of a real-world stressful event on participants' state level of anxiety was reduced by ABM training.

Attention Bias Modification in Pediatric Populations

The evidence discussed above shows that ABM training is a promising new treatment for reducing internalizing problems, particularly anxiety, in adults. However, internalizing problems typically emerge during childhood, and potentially fruitful new applications of ABM training are focused on the treatment of childhood anxiety and the prevention of later anxiety onset in children at risk. ABM may be particularly useful in children, who may not have fully developed the cognitive skills required to be successful in traditional cognitive behavioral therapy [O'Toole & Dennis, 2013; Pérez-Edgar et al., 2013]. While the currently available research on ABM in children is limited, it does suggest that this is a promising direction for attention training research and that more studies in pediatric populations are needed.

Eldar et al. [2008] conducted an early study of ABM in nonanxious youths and found that training toward threat increased vigilance to threat and stress-induced anxiety, but training away from threat did not have either effect. The lack of an effect of training away from threat might be explained by the fact that the sample (healthy, nonanxious youths) was not the intended or typical target for ABM treatment. Indeed, in recent years, studies of ABM in children with anxiety or subclinical internalizing symptomatology have yielded more promising results.

Rozenman et al. [2011] reported on the impact of ABM training in a case series of 16 children and adolescents diagnosed with anxiety disorder. All patients underwent active ABM training for 12 sessions of 160 trails (15–20 min) over 4 weeks, with standard face pairs displaying neutral and threatening (i.e., anger and disgust), to train attention away from threat. The study found that ABM was feasible in youths and may indeed be effective, as 12 of the 16 patients no longer met diagnostic criteria after treatment. However, the lack of a control group was a significant limitation.

Following this case series studies have shifted to the gold-standard of randomized controlled trials and have demonstrated the effectiveness of ABM in children. For example, in pediatric anxiety disorder, 4 weekly sessions of face (neutral/threat) ABM training away from threat were shown to be more effective in reducing anxiety symptoms than placebo tasks without training or with both neutral faces [Eldar et al., 2012]. Another randomized controlled trial by Bar-Haim et al. [2012] tested 34 high-anxious 10-year-olds who completed four sessions over two weeks of ABM or placebo task. The authors found that, relative to the control group, the ABM group showed significantly faster disengagement from threat post-training, and significantly less state anxiety in response to stress induction (being videotaped while attempting to solve difficult puzzles). Our lab is currently in the midst of a randomized control ABM trial with 9- to 12-year-olds high in behavioral inhibition. Although preliminary, our data also suggest that self-reported anxiety decreases after 4 weeks of ABM, relative to placebo controls.

Neural and Psychophysiological Correlates of ABM

The specific psychological mechanisms by which attention bias modification training tasks exert their effects on attention processes remain to be fully understood [Fox & Pine, 2012; Shechner et al., 2012]. For example, Heeren et al. [2012] tested variants of dot-probe-like ABM tasks to narrow in on which aspect of the task is the active ingredient. Participants were randomly assigned to receive one of four ABM tasks, which were altered to disentangle potential causal mechanisms by training just: (a) re-engagement to nonthreat, (b) disengagement from threat, (c) disengagement from threat and reengagement to nonthreat, or (d) neither (placebo). The study revealed that only training to disengage from threat reduced anxiety, while re-engagement to nonthreat had no effects by itself. These findings are in agreement with the available neuroimaging literature [Britton, Lissek, Grillon, Norcross & Pine, 2011; Telzer et al., 2008]. Thus, it seems that difficulty in disengaging from threat may be a crucial process in the maintenance of anxiety over time, and that ABM may act by altering this underlying developmental tether. Additional basic studies of this sort will be important going forward to hone in on the specific mechanisms underlying anxiety-related attention biases and to better target attention bias modification treatments.

Building on what is known about the fronto-limbic neural processes underlying attention bias and threat processing [Pine, 2007], researchers have begun to hypothesize about and explore the impacts of ABM training on neural functioning. According to Fox and Pine [2012], ABM may work at the neural level by strengthening vlPFC inhibitory control over amygdala and limbic system functioning. Repeated training of attention toward neutral stimuli in an ABM task may build the neural disposition (encoded in vlPFC) to deploy attention toward nonthreatening information, so that in future trials (perhaps both experimental and real-world) the individual is more capable of inhibiting the bias to attend to threat, thereby stemming the cycle of negative information processing before it starts.

Research linking attention bias to threat with vlPFC and amygdala function [Monk et al., 2006,

2008; Pine, 2007] combined with the evidence that ABM modifies attention bias to threat [Hakamata et al., 2010], support the suggestion that ABM likely has impacts on this frontolimbic network. Furthermore, one fMRI study examined the impact of ABM training on neural functioning in 29 young, healthy adults [Browning, Holmes, Murphy, Goodwin, & Harmer, 2009]. Following the procedures of MacLeod et al. [2002], Browning et al. [2009] trained half of the participants away from threat and half toward threat in one brief training session. Immediately after testing, participants were then placed in the scanner to perform an unrelated face-processing task. Those trained away from threat showed greater dorsolateral PFC activation to angry versus neutral faces than participants trained toward threat. Although the activation was dorsal, rather than ventral lateral PFC, this is likely due to the difference in task used in the scanner.

As with studies of attention bias, ERP studies can supplement our understanding of the potential functional mechanisms of ABM. As noted, it has been assumed that ABM impacts anxiety by improving attentional control [Fox & Pine, 2012], allowing individuals to break the early bias to attend to threat. If this was the case, then changes in anxiety-related behaviors fueled by changes in attentional control should be reflected not only in reported levels of anxiety, but also in neurobiological and physiological measures. The few studies examining this question have found support for this hypothesis.

An ERP study with anxious individuals [Eldar & Bar-Haim, 2010] found that ABM modified later attentional processes (N2, P2, and P3), reflecting more effortful or endogenous attentional mechanisms. However, an ERP study with nonanxious individuals [Dennis, O'Toole & DeCicco, 2013] found that ABM altered earlier components of attention (P1). This implies that ABM might modify attention through different processes between anxious and nonanxious individuals.

Other physiological methods have also shown differences after ABM. For example, Heeren et al. [2012], in a modification of ABM, found that individuals with social phobia who trained attention towards nonthreatening stimuli (i.e., happy faces) showed reduced skin conductance response towards stress after training. Similarly, Dandeneau et al. [2007] found that individuals after ABM exhibited decreased cortisol release during a stressful task. Our preliminary data also suggest that ABM may decrease levels of right frontal EEG asymmetry in behaviorally inhibited children. Together, this corpus of evidence suggests that ABM modifies not only the implicit attentional bias towards threat, but also changes physiological and neurobiological aspects of attention, attention control, and emotional responses towards threatening stimuli.

Future Directions in the Study of Attention and Anxiety

Basic and clinical research on the modification of attention biases has yielded exciting results, with the promise to add a low-cost, low-risk tool to the anxiety treatment toolbox. However, this research is in its infancy and pressing questions remain. While some work has begun to dig into the basic mechanisms underlying the seeming success of ABM [Rothbart et al., 2011; Shechner et al., 2012], it is crucial to further explore the psychological and biological mechanism involved in order to fully understand the impacts, appropriate use cases, and potential side effects of ABM.

As it is, a long series of questions remain unanswered. They include the following: What are the mechanisms by which ABM may act to impact anxiety? How long do the effects of ABM persist? How broad a 'reach' does ABM have in impacting the deep-seated, problematic behavioral patterns that are characteristic of clinical anxiety? Can temperamentally at-risk youths be targeted for intervention, using ABM as an inoculation tool? Finally, how do the effects of ABM interact with the normative developmental trajectories of attention?

Our laboratory is one of many now working to address these questions, examining the impact of attention biases and ABM on the cognitive, behavioral and neural correlates of anxiety and temperamental risk. Manipulating attention acts as one of the earliest emerging self-regulatory tools available to children [Posner, Rothbart, Sheese & Voelker, 2012]. The reviewed studies suggest that attention biases play an early developmental role in modulating the risk for anxiety. Thus, future studies will need to focus systematically on the ways in which attention mechanisms and socio-emotional behavior develop hand-in-hand over the course of childhood. The information gained may allow us to increase our ability to intervene at the earliest signs of vulnerability by targeting one of the most pervasive functional mechanisms of risk.

Acknowledgement

Support for manuscript preparation was provided by grants from the National Institutes of Health (MH# 094633) and The Pennsylvania State University Social Science Research Institute (Level II Grant) to Koraly Pérez-Edgar.

References

Almas, A.N., Phillips, D.A., Henderson, H.A., Hane, A.A., Degnan, K.A., Moas, O.L., & Fox, N.A. (2011). The relations between infant negative reactivity, non-maternal childcare, and children's interactions with familiar and unfamiliar peers. *Social Development, 20*, 718–740.

Amir, N., Beard, C., Burns, M., & Bomyea, J. (2009). Attention modification program in individuals with Generalized Anxiety Disorder. *Journal of Abnormal Psychology, 109*, 28–33.

Amir, N., Beard, C., Taylor, C.T., Klumpp, H., Elias, J., Burns, M., & Chen, X. (2009). Attention training in individuals with generalized social phobia: A randomized controlled trial. *Journal of Consulting and Clinical Psychology, 77*, 961–973.

Amir, N., Bomyea, J., & Beard, C. (2010). The effect of single-session interpretation modification on attention bias in socially anxious individuals. *Journal of Anxiety Disorders, 24*, 178–182.

Bar-Haim, Y. (2010). Research review: attention bias modification (ABM): A novel treatment for anxiety disorders. *Journal of Child Psychology & Psychiatry, 51*, 859–870.

Bar-Haim, Y., Lamy, D., Pergamin, L., Bakermans-Kranenburg, M., & van IJzendoorn, M. (2007). Threat-related attentional bias in anxious and nonanxious individuals: A meta-analytic study. *Psychological Bulletin, 133*, 1–24.

Bar-Haim, Y., Morag, I., & Glickman, S. (2012). Training anxious children to disengage attention from threat: A randomized controlled trial. *Journal of Child Psychology & Psychiatry, 52*, 861–869.

Beevers, C.G., Gibb, B., McGeary, J.E., & Miller, I.W. (2007). Serotonin transporter genetic variation and biased attention for emotional word stimuli among psychiatric inpatients. *Journal of Abnormal Psychology, 116*, 208–212.

Biederman, J., Faraone, S.V., Hirshfeld-Becker, D.R., Friedman, D., Robin, J.A., & Rosenbaum, J.F. (2001). Patterns of psychopathology and dysfunction in high-risk children of parents with panic disorder and major depression. *American Journal of Psychiatry, 158*, 49–57.

Britton, J.C., Bar-Haim, Y., Carver, F.W., Holroyd, T., Norcross, M.A., Detloff, A., & Pine, D.S. (2012). Isolating neural components of threat bias in pediatric anxiety. *Journal of Child Psychology & Psychiatry, 53*, 678–686.

Britton, J.C., Bar-Haim, Y., Clementi, M.A., Sankin, L.S., Chen, G., Shechner, T., & Pine, D.S. (2013). Training-associated changes and stability of attention bias in youth: Implications for Attention Bias Modification Treatment for pediatric anxiety. *Developmental Cognitive Neuroscience, 4*, 52–64.

Britton, J.C., Lissek, S., Grillon, C., Norcross, M.A., & Pine, D.S. (2011). Development of anxiety: the role of threat appraisal and fear learning. *Depression and Anxiety, 28*, 5–17. doi: 10.1002/da.20733.

Browning, M., Holmes, E.A., Murphy, S.E., Goodwin, G.M., & Harmer, C.J. (2009). Lateral prefrontal cortex mediates the cognitive modification of attentional bias. *Biological Psychiatry, 67*, 919–925.

Buss, K.A., & Keil, E.J. (2013). Temperamental risk factors for pediatric anxiety disorders. In R.A. Vasa & A.K. Roy (Eds.), *Pediatric Anxiety Disorders: A Clinical Guide* (pp. 47–68). New York, Springer.

Chronis-Tuscano, A., Degnan, K., Pine, D., Perez-Edgar, K., Henderson, H., Diaz, Y., & Fox, N.A. (2009). Stable behavioral inhibition during infancy and early childhood predicts the development of anxiety disorders in adolescence. *Journal of the American Academy of Child & Adolescent Psychiatry, 48*, 928–935.

Coplan, R.J., Rubin, K.H., Fox, N.A., Calkins, S.D., & Stewart, S.L. (1994). Being alone, playing alone, and acting alone: distinguishing among reticence and passive and active solitude in young children. *Child Development, 65*, 129–137.

Crick, N.R., & Dodge, K.A. (1994). A review and reformulation of social information-processing mechanisms in children's social adjustment. *Psychological Bulletin, 115*, 74–101.

Dandeneau, S.D., Baldwin, M.W., Baccus, J.R., Sakellaropoulo, M., & Pruessner, J.C. (2007). Cutting stress off at the pass: Reducing vigilance and responsiveness to social threat by manipulating attention. *Journal of Personality and Social Psychology, 93*, 651–666. doi: 10.1037/0022-3514.93.4.651.

Degnan, K.A., Almas, A.N., & Fox, N.A. (2010). Temperament and the environment in the etiology of childhood anxiety. *Journal of Child Psychology and Psychiatry, 51*, 497–517.

Degnan, K.A., & Fox, N.A. (2007). Behavioral inhibition and anxiety disorders: Multiple levels of a resilience process. *Development and Psychopathology, 19*, 729–746.

Dennis, T.A., O'Toole, L., & DeCicco, J. (2013). Emotion regulation from the perspective of developmental neuroscience: What, Where, When, and Why. In K. Barrett (Ed.), *The handbook of self-regulatory processes*. New York: Taylor & Francis.

Eldar, S., Apter, A., Lotan, D., Pérez-Edgar, K., Naim, R., Fox, N.A., & Bar-Haim, Y. (2012). Attention bias modification in clinically anxious children: A randomized control trial. *American Journal of Psychiatry, 169*, 213–222.

Eldar, S., & Bar-Haim, Y. (2010). Neural plasticity in response to attention training in anxiety. *Psychological Medicine, 40*, 667–677.

Eldar, S., Ricon, T., & Bar-Haim, Y. (2008). Plasticity in attention: Implications for stress response in children. *Behaviour Research & Therapy, 46*, 450–461.

Eldar, S., Yankelevitch, R., Lamy, D., & Bar-Haim, Y. (2010). Enhanced neural reactivity and selective attention to threat in anxiety. *Biological Psychology, 85*, 252–257.

Fox, E., Ridgewell, A., & Ashwin, C. (2009). Looking on the bright side: biased attention and the human serotonin transporter gene. *Proceedings of the Royal Society B, Biological Sciences, 276*, 1747–1751.

Fox, N.A., Henderson, H.A., Pérez-Edgar, K., & White, L. (2008). The biology of temperament: An integrative approach. In C. Nelson & M. Luciana (Eds.), *The Handbook of Developmental Cognitive Neuroscience* (pp. 839–854). Cambridge, MA: MIT Press.

Fox, N.A., & Pine, D.S. (2012). Temperament and the emergence of anxiety disorders. *Journal of the American Academy of Child and Adolescent Psychiatry, 51*, 125–128.

Fox, N.A., Rubin, K.H., Calkins, S.D., Marshall, T.R., Coplan, R.J., Porges, S.W., & Stewart, S. (1995). Frontal activation asymmetry and social competence at four years of age. *Child Development, 66*, 1771–1784.

Garcia Coll, C., Kagan, J., & Reznick, J.S. (1984). Behavioral inhibition in young children. *Child Development, 55*, 1005–1019.

Gibb, B.E., Benas, J.S., Grassia, M., & McGeary, J. (2009). Children's attentional biases and 5-HTTLPR genotype: Potential mechanisms linking mother and child depression. [Article]. *Journal of Clinical Child and Adolescent Psychology, 38*, 415–426.

Hakamata, Y., Lissek, S., Bar-Haim, Y., Britton, J.C., Fox, N.A., Leibenluft, E., & Pine, D.S. (2010). Attention Bias Modification Treatment: A meta-analysis towards the establishment of novel treatment for anxiety. *Biological Psychiatry, 68*, 982–990.

Hardee, J., Benson, B., Bar-Haim, Y., Mogg, K., Bradley, B.P., Chen, G., Britton, J., Ernst, M., Fox, N.A., Pine, D.S., & Pérez-Edgar, K. (2013). Patterns of neural connectivity during an attention bias task moderate associations between early childhood temperament and internalizing symptoms in young adulthood. *Biological Psychiatry, 74*, 273–279.

Heeren, A., Reese, H.E., McNally, R.J., & Philippot, P. (2012). Attention training toward and away from threat in social phobia: Effects on subjective, behavioral, and physiological measures of anxiety. *Behaviour Research and Therapy, 50*, 30–39.

Helfinstein, S.M., White, L.K., Bar-Haim, Y., & Fox, N.A. (2008). Affective primes suppress attention bias to threat in socially anxious individuals. *Behaviour Research & Therapy, 46*, 799–810.

Kagan, J. (2012). The biography of behavioral inhibition. In M. Zentner & R.L. Shiner (Eds.), *Handbook of Temperament* (pp. 69–82). New York: Guilford Press.

Kagan, J., Reznick, J.S., & Snidman, N. (1987). The physiology and psychology of behavioral inhibition in children. *Child Development, 58*, 1459–1473.

Kagan, J., Snidman, N., McManis, M., & Woodward, S. (2001). Temperamental contributions to the affect family of anxiety. *The Psychiatric Clinics of North America, 24*, 677–688.

LoBue, V. (2013). What are we so afraid of? How early attention shapes our most common fears. *Child Development Perspectives, 7*, 38–42. doi: 10.1111/cdep.12012.

Lonigan, C., & Vasey, M. (2009). Negative affectivity, effortful control, and attention to threat-relevant stimuli. *Journal of Abnormal Child Psychology, 37*, 387–399.

MacLeod, C., & Mathews, A. (2012). Cognitive bias modification approaches to anxiety. *Annual Review of Clinical Psychology, 8*, 189–217.

MacLeod, C., Mathews, A., & Tata, P. (1986). Attentional bias in emotional disorders. *Journal of Abnormal Psychology, 95*, 15–20.

MacLeod, C., Rutherford, E., Campbell, L., Ebsworthy, G., & Holker, L. (2002). Selective attention and emotional vulnerability: Assessing the causal basis of their association through the experimental manipulation of attentional bias. *Journal of Abnormal Psychology, 111*, 107–123.

Mathews, A., & MacLeod, C. (1994). Cognitive approaches to emotion and emotional disorders. *Annual Review of Psychology, 45*, 25–50.

Mathews, A., & MacLeod, C. (2002). Induced processing biases have causal effects on anxiety. *Cognition and Emotion, 16*, 331–354.

Mogg, K., Bradley, B.P., De Bono, J., & Painter, M. (1997). Time course of attentional bias for threat information in non-clinical anxiety. *Behaviour Research & Therapy, 35*, 297–303.

Mogg, K., Bradley, B.P., Miles, F., & Dixon, R. (2004). Time course of attentional bias for threat scenes: Testing the vigilance-avoidance hypothesis. *Cognition and Emotion, 18*, 689–700.

Monk, C.S., Nelson, E.E., McClure, E.B., Mogg, K., Bradley, B.P., Leibenluft, E., & Pine, D.S. (2006). Ventrolateral prefrontal cortex activation and attention bias in responsive to angry faces in adolescents with generalized anxiety disorder. *American Journal of Psychiatry, 163*, 1091–1097.

Monk, C.S., Telzer, E.H., Mogg, K., Bradley, B.P., Mai, X., Louro, H.M.C., & Pine, D.S. (2008). Amygdala and ventrolateral prefrontal cortex activation to masked angry faces in children and adolescents with generalized anxiety disorder. *Archives of General Psychiatry, 65*, 568–576.

O'Toole, L., & Dennis, T.A. (2013). Neurophysiological Correlates of Attention Bias Modification for Anxiety in Adults and Children: Individual Differences and Prediction of Treatment Response. Paper presented at the 25th Association for Psychological Science Annual Convention, Washington, DC.

Oldfield, R. (1971). The assessment and analysis of handedness: the Edinburgh inventory. *Neuropsychologia, 9*, 97–113.

Penkunas, M.J., & Coss, R.G. (2013). A comparison of rural and urban Indian children's visual detection of threatening and nonthreatening animals. *Developmental Science, 16*, 463–475.

Pérez-Edgar, K., Bar-Haim, Y., McDermott, J.M., Chronis-Tuscano, A., Pine, D.S., & Fox, N.A. (2010). Attention biases to threat and behavioral inhibition in early childhood shape adolescent social withdrawal. *Emotion, 10*, 349–357.

Pérez-Edgar, K., Bar-Haim, Y., McDermott, J.M., Gorodetsky, E., Hodgkinson, C.A., Goldman, D., & Fox, N.A. (2010). Variations in the serotonin transporter gene are linked to heightened attention bias to threat. *Biological Psychology, 83*, 269–271.

Pérez-Edgar, K., & Fox, N.A. (2005). Temperament and anxiety disorders. *Child and Adolescent Psychiatric Clinics of North America, 14*, 681–706.

Pérez-Edgar, K., McDermott, J.M., Korelitz, K., Degnan, K.A., Curby, T.W., Pine, D.S., & Fox, N.A. (2010). Patterns of sustained attention in infancy shape the developmental trajectory of social behavior from toddlerhood through adolescence. *Developmental Psychology, 46*, 1723–1730.

Pérez-Edgar, K., Reeb-Sutherland, B.C., McDermott, J.M., White, L.K., Henderson, H.A., Degnan, K.A., & Fox, N.A. (2011). Attention biases to threat link behavioral inhibition to social withdrawal over time in very young children. *Journal of Abnormal Child Psychology, 39*, 885–895.

Pérez-Edgar, K., Taber-Thomas, B.C., Thai, N., Morales, S., & Danilo, C. (2013). Electrophysiological and Neural Correlates of Attention Bias Modification in Behaviorally Inhibited Children. Paper presented at the 25th Association for Psychological Science Annual Convention, Washington, DC.

Pine, D.S. (2007). Research review: A neuroscience framework for pediatric anxiety disorders. *Journal of Child Psychology and Psychiatry, 48*, 631–648.

Pine, D.S., Helfinstein, S.M., Bar-Haim, Y., Nelson, E., & Fox, N.A. (2009). Challenges in developing novel treatments for childhood disorders: Lessons from research on anxiety. *Neuropsychopharmacology, 34*, 213–228.

Posner, M.I., Rothbart, M.K., Sheese, B.E., & Voelker, P. (2012). Control networks and neuromodulators of early development. *Developmental Psychology, 48*, 827–835.

Rothbart, M.K. (2012). Advances in temperament: History, concepts, and measures. In M. Zentner & R.L. Shiner (Eds.), *Handbook of temperament* (pp. 3–20). New York: Guilford Press.

Rothbart, M.K., Ahadi, S., & Evans, D. (2000). Temperament and personality: Origins and outcomes. *Journal of Personality and Social Psychology, 78*, 122–135.

Rothbart, M.K., Sheese, B.E., Rueda, M.R., & Posner, M.I. (2011). Developing mechanisms of self-regulation in early life. *Emotion Review, 3*, 207–213.

Roy, A.K., Vasa, R.A., Bruck, M., Mogg, K., Bradley, B.P., Sweeney, M., & Pine, D.S. (2008). Attention bias toward threat in pediatric anxiety disorders. *Journal of the American Academy of Child & Adolescent Psychiatry, 47*, 1189–1196.

Rozenman, M., Weersing, V.R., & Amir, N. (2011). A case series of attention modification in clinically anxious youths. *Behaviour Research and Therapy, 49*, 324–330.

Rubin, K., Chen, X., & Hymel, S. (1993). Socioemotional characteristics of withdrawn and aggressive children. *Merrill-Palmer Quarterly, 39*, 518–534.

Schmidt, L.A., Fox, N.A., Rubin, K.H., Sternberg, E.M., Gold, P.W., Smith, C.C., & Schulkin, J. (1997). Behavioral and neuroendocrine responses in shy children. *Developmental Psychobiology, 30*, 127–140.

Schmidt, L.A., Fox, N.A., Schulkin, J., & Gold, P.W. (1999). Behavioral and psychophysiological correlates of self-presentation in temperamentally shy children. *Developmental Psychobiology, 35*, 119–135.

Schmidt, N.B., Richey, J., Buckner, J., & Timpano, K. (2009). Attention training for Generalized Social Anxiety Disorder. *Journal of Abnormal Psychology, 118*, 5–14.

See, J., MacLeod, C., & Bridle, R. (2009). The reduction of anxiety vulnerability through the modification of attentional bias: A real-world study using a home-based cognitive bias modification procedure. *Journal of Abnormal Psychology, 109*, 65–75.

Shechner, T., Britton, J.C., Pérez-Edgar, K., Bar-Haim, Y., Ernst, M., Fox, N.A., & Pine, D.S. (2012). Attention biases, anxiety, and development: Toward or away from threats or rewards? *Depression & Anxiety, 29*, 282–294.

Shechner, T., Jarcho, J.M., Britton, J.C., Leibenluft, E., Pine, D.S., & Nelson, E.E. (2013). Attention bias of anxious youth during extended exposure of emotional face pairs: an eye-tracking study. *Depression & Anxiety, 30*, 14–21. doi: 10.1002/da.21986.

Susa, G., Pitică, I., Benga, O., & Miclea, M. (2012). The self regulatory effect of attentional control in modulating the relationship between attentional biases toward threat and anxiety symptoms in children. *Cognition & Emotion, 26*, 1069–1083.

Telzer, E.H., Mogg, K., Bradley, B.P., Mai, X., Ernst, M., Pine, D.S., & Monk, C.S. (2008). Relationship between trait anxiety, prefrontal cortex, and attention bias to angry faces in children and adolescents. *Biological Psychology, 79*, 216–222.

Todd, R.M., Cunningham, W.A., Anderson, A.K., & Thompson, E. (2012). Affect-biased attention as emotion regulation. *Trends in Cognitive Sciences, 16*, 365–372.

Tottenham, N., Tanaka, J., Leon, A., McCarry, T., Nurse, M., Hare, T., & Nelson, C. (2009). The NimStim set of facial expressions: Judgments from untrained research participants. *Psychiatry Research, 168*, 242–249.

Waters, A.M., Bradley, B.P., & Mogg, K. (in press). Biased attention to threat in paediatric anxiety disorders (generalized anxiety disorder, social phobia, specific phobia, separation anxiety disorder) as a function of 'distress' versus 'fear' diagnostic categorization. *Psychological Medicine.*

Waters, A.M., Henry, J., Mogg, K., Bradley, B.P., & Pine, D.S. (2010). Attentional bias towards angry faces in childhood anxiety disorders. *Journal of Behavior Therapy and Experimental Psychiatry, 41*, 158–164.

Waters, A.M., Mogg, K., Bradley, B.P., & Pine, D.S. (2008). Attentional bias for emotional faces in children with generalized anxiety disorder. *Journal of the American Academy of Child & Adolescent Psychiatry, 47*, 435–442.

Wells, A., & Matthews, G. (1996). Modeling cognition in emotional disorder: The S-REF model. *Behaviour Research and Therapy, 34*, 881–888.

White, L.K., Helfinstein, S.M., & Fox, N.A. (2010). Temperamental Factors Associated with the Acquisition of Information Processing Biases and Anxiety. In J.A. Hadwin & A.P. Field (Eds.), *Information Processing Biases and Anxiety: A Developmental Perspective* (pp. 233–252). Chichester, UK: John Wiley & Sons.

Williams, L.R., Degnan, K.A., Pérez-Edgar, K., Henderson, H.A., Rubin, K.H., Pine, D.S., & Fox, N.A. (2009). Impact of behavioral inhibition and parenting style on internalizing and externalizing problems from early childhood through adolescence. *Journal of Abnormal Child Psychology, 37*, 1063–1075.

Koraly Pérez-Edgar
Department of Psychology, The Pennsylvania State University
111 Moore Bldg
University Park, PA 16802-3106 (USA)
E-Mail kxp24@psu.edu

Hansen Lagattuta K (ed): Children and Emotion. New Insights into Developmental Affective Sciences.
Contrib Hum Dev. Basel, Karger, 2014, vol 26, pp 57–66 (DOI: 10.1159/000354353)

Emotional Competence and Social Relations

Elizabeth A. Lemerise[a] · Bridgette D. Harper[b]

[a]Department of Psychology, Western Kentucky University, Bowling Green, Ky., and
[b]Department of Psychology, Auburn University at Montgomery, Montgomery, Ala., USA

Abstract

Models of emotional competence are briefly reviewed and a working definition of emotional competence is offered. We address how emotional competence is related to social relations in two ways. First, we review research on how the skills of emotional competence develop in the context of parent-child relationships. Then, we discuss how the emotional competence skills acquired in parent-child relationships help children to negotiate the broader world of peers. In addition, we discuss obstacles children may experience in developing emotional competence as well as preventive interventions designed to address those challenges.

A number of researchers have offered definitions and models of emotional competence [Crick & Dodge, 1994; Halberstadt, Denham & Dunsmore, 2001; Lemerise & Arsenio, 2000; Mayer & Salovey, 1997; Saarni, 1999]; these models are reviewed in order to identify points of intersection and to synthesize a working definition of emotional competence. We then address how emotional competence is related to social relations. First, we describe how emotional competence develops in a relational context, with a discussion of how infants' and children's early relationships with caregivers contribute to the development of emotional competence. As children develop, relationships with siblings, peers, and others provide additional relational contexts for the development of the skills that comprise emotional competence, and skills acquired in the context of the parent-child relationship help children negotiate these new relational contexts. In other words, not only do social relations provide a context for the development of the component skills of emotional competence, but individual differences in emotional competence can affect the nature of an individual's social relations outside the parent-child relationship. We focus on the preschool years as this is a time of rapid development of key emotional competence skills, making it an intriguing age period for examining how individual differences in emotional competence impact social relations.

What Is Emotional Competence?

Some theorists frame emotional competence as a specific intelligence (i.e. emotional intelligence, EI) [Mayer, Salovey & Caruso, 2004; Mayer, Salovey, Caruso & Sitarenios, 2001] that is heavily influenced by biology and related to general intelligence. EI allows people to reason about emotions and to use emotions and emotion regulation to enhance their general intelligence and cognitive abilities. Theorists adhering to this perspective focus on identifying and measuring the biologically based individual differences in EI ability and the subsequent links between EI and overall intelligence. Thus, being highly emotionally intelligent means one can use these abilities successfully to monitor one's own and others' emotions and to use this information to guide goal-oriented behavior [Mayer et al., 2000, 2004].

Another body of research emphasizes the functional role emotions play in helping people adapt to their environments [Denham, 1998; Saarni, Mumme & Campos, 1998]. Although these theorists acknowledge the existence of biological influences on emotional competence, they also contend that learning, experience, and socialization of emotions all work to influence these biological substrates. Therefore, the social context bears heavily on the successful development of emotional competence. Saarni [1990, 1997, 1999] argued that achieving emotional competence requires mastery of eight skills including learning to become aware of your own and others' emotions, using emotion language to express emotion, and displaying empathy [see Saarni, 1990, for a full review]. Each skill builds on subsequent skills, and the skills, when mastered, ultimately lead to the ability to exhibit emotional competence even during highly-charged situations. Saarni contends that people demonstrate emotional competence when they exhibit self-efficacy while experiencing an emotion-eliciting event.

Crick and Dodge [1994] proposed a six-step social information processing (SIP) model that outlines the various steps of reaching socially competent or incompetent decisions. In steps one and two, relevant cues are encoded and interpreted; in step three, goals are clarified; in steps four and five, responses are accessed, evaluated, and one is chosen; finally, in step six, the chosen response is enacted. Although this model provides a detailed description of how children interpret and react to social cues, it does not afford much attention to emotion and how emotion could directly and indirectly influence each step of this process. Lemerise and Arsenio [2000] proposed an integrated model of social information processing which addresses how emotion processes such as emotionality/temperament, emotion regulation, and moods/background emotions influence each step of Crick and Dodge's [1994] model of SIP. In particular, Lemerise and Arsenio [2000] highlight the importance of affective cues from peers and the affective nature of the relationship with peers for encoding social cues, interpreting cues, clarifying goals, and ultimately deciding what to do. Even this updated model, however, neglects to consider how children learn to successfully send affective cues and how children learn to understand and manage their own affective signals.

Another approach frames emotional competence in terms of affective social competence (ASC) [Halberstadt et al., 2001]. Rather than focusing on particular skills or steps, this theory is unique in that it highlights the importance of three previously overlooked components of emotion communication: sending emotional messages, receiving emotional messages, and experiencing emotional messages. Each component is dependent upon the development of four abilities, awareness of one's own emotions, identification of others' emotions, the ability to work within a social context, and the ability to manage and regulate emotions. To be competent affective communicators, children must be able to participate successfully in each component. Similar to Saarni [1997], ASC theorists also contend that effective communicators understand the role that partners and the social context play in emotional experiences; however, ASC theorists point out that skilled communicators not only respond emotionally to the here and now, but they also take into account past experiences and future goals when interacting with a partner.

Even though each theory focuses on a unique aspect of emotional competence, there is consensus across the theories about the necessary skills to become emotionally competent. The first point of intersection is what we will call emotional awareness and identification. For example, Mayer and Salovey [1997] point out that the first ability of EI is perceiving (being aware of) and appraising (or identifying) your own and others' emotions, and ability three of their theory encompasses recognizing and interpreting emotions in others [see Mayer & Salovey, 1997, for a full review of this theory]. Similar to this contention, Saarni [1997] argues that being aware of one's emotional state and recognizing other's emotions are the first two skills needed for emotional competence. In addition, the first two steps of SIP theory [Crick & Dodge, 1994; Lemerise & Arsenio, 2000] highlight the importance of encoding internal and external emotional cues (i.e., becoming aware of emotions) and the correct interpretation of these cues. According to these theorists, it is during steps two and three of SIP that causal attributions and evaluation of goals takes place. Halberstadt et al. [2001] proposed an ASC model which centers emotional awareness and interpretation around three components; sending, receiving (awareness), and experiencing (interpreting) affective messages.

Why are emotion awareness and interpretation key elements across all theories? Correctly recognizing emotions in the self and others leads to a clearer understanding of emotions as well as a more accurate understanding of the social situations associated with those emotions. Awareness of emotions and interpretation of emotions also initiates the correct usage of emotion language, skill three of Saarni's [1997] theory. Emotion language is critical in allowing children to let others know how they are feeling and in gaining feedback about their emotional states. In addition, being emotionally aware allows children to begin to use contextual cues to link causes and consequences of emotion which also contributes to children's understanding of social situations [Denham, 1998; Saarni et al., 1998]. Clearly then, being aware of and correctly identifying your own and others' emotions is of primary importance for the development of emotional competence. In addition, being aware of and correctly identifying emotions contributes to successful emotion regulation, the second key point of intersection among these theories.

Saarni [1990, 1999], Mayer and Salovey [1997], Crick and Dodge [1994], and Lemerise and Arsenio [2000] specifically highlight the need for emotion or arousal regulation, broadly defined as the ability to generate and engage in appropriate coping responses (attentional, cognitive, and/or behavioral) during an emotion-eliciting event [Trentacosta & Shaw, 2009]. Saarni [1990] labels this ability as *adaptive coping*, whereas Mayer and Salovey [1997] term this ability *emotion regulation*. SIP theorists [Crick & Dodge, 1994; Lemerise & Arsenio, 2000] view this capacity as *arousal regulation*, whereas ASC theorists [Halberstadt et al., 2001] identify management of emotions as key to influencing each component of affective social competence.

No matter how it is labeled, regulation of emotion is important to each theory because regulating emotions allows for the successful monitoring, evaluating, and modifying of emotional reactions to allow ultimate goal obtainment. In Mayer and Salovey's [1997] model, the ability to generate emotions to assist thoughts influences children's self-awareness of both positive and negative emotions and can lead to self-monitoring to calm down in provocative situations (ability four of their model). Saarni [1990] contends that self-regulation ultimately leads to children understanding their own and other's emotional states better. Achieving self-regulation both increases a child's empathic understanding of others and ultimately a feeling of emotional self-efficacy [Saarni, 1990, 1999]. SIP theory argues that with proper regulation, children should be able to generate more response options [Lemerise & Arsenio, 2000] in relation to emotion-eliciting events. Emotion regulation is critical because the more responses a child is able to access during an emotion-eliciting event, the better the chance the child will behaviorally enact an appropriate response. If a child is unable to control the intensity of emotions, however, then generating and evaluating possible responses (steps four and five) suffers, and the likelihood that the child will respond inappropriately increases (step six) [Crick & Dodge, 1994; Lemerise & Arsenio, 2000].

Taken together, these theories suggest that emotional competence involves developing skills in emotion awareness and interpretation, emotion regulation, and enacting appropriate behavioral responses during emotion-eliciting events. In addition, these skills do not emerge in isolation from one another but rather proficiency in one area influences development in other areas. For example, if a child mislabels sadness as anger, this mislabeling could lead to deficiencies in emotion regulation. We discuss how the skills of emotional competence develop below.

Emotional Competence Develops in a Relational Context

If emotional competence involves the ability to accurately perceive and identify emotions, regulate emotional arousal, and enact appropriate behavioral responses during emotion-eliciting events, how do these skills develop in young children? Although biological factors such as temperament play a role [Thompson, 2009] many of the components of emotional competence develop within the context of relationships [Waters et al., 2010]. For toddlers and preschoolers, the earliest and most influential relationships for emotional development are those they share with their parents. Parent-child attachment and parental direct and indirect emotion socialization are two key influences on children's subsequent emotional competence [Thompson & Meyer, 2007; Waters et al., 2010].

Quality parent-child relationships characterized by high levels of warmth, security, and reciprocity are critical in the development of children's emotional competence [Denham, 1998; Denham, Renwick-DeBardi & Hewes, 1994]. These factors work together to help children navigate and learn about their emotional worlds. For example, preschool children involved in mutually warm relationships develop a higher level of trust with their caregivers, and they are much more likely to share their thoughts and feelings about their personal experiences with their caregivers [Waters, Kondo-Ikemura, Posada & Richters, 1991], a key factor in learning how to both identify emotions and to understand the causes and consequences of emotions. Warm relationships also lead to a sense of security, an important factor in gaining a child's willingness to cooperate with and to be socialized by their caregivers [Kochanska, 1995; Thompson, 1998]. In addition, preschoolers who are securely attached to their caregivers tend to get along better and form more intimate relationships with peers and other adults [Bretherton & Munholland, 1999; Thompson, 1998]. Parent-child relationships marked with high levels of security also tend to be high in mutual reciprocity, a kind of social obligation where prosocial behaviors (e.g., acts of kindness) are expected to be reciprocated. In these types of relationships, parents show more empathy for their children and use less coercive forms of discipline; in return, their children cooperate more with parental requests and demonstrate higher levels of empathy within the parent-child relationship and peer relationships [Kochanska, 2002; Kochanska & Murray, 2000; Laible & Thompson, 2000].

There are two primary ways that parents directly socialize children's emotional development: *coaching* and *contingencies* (validating or punishing emotions). By correctly labeling children's emotions and teaching children appropriate coping strategies, parents contribute to both children's emotion knowledge and regulation [Gottman, Katz & Hooven, 1997]. Correctly labeling emotions shows that parents are accepting of children's emotions and helps children learn to discriminate between emotional states. Coaching then teaches young children how to cope with their emotions and what to say and do in emotion-eliciting situations, including how to express these feelings appropriately [Denham, 1998; Gottman et al., 1997; Laible & Panfile, 2009; Thompson, 2006]. For example, children often express fear about getting an injection. Parents who validate emotions and coach coping strategies might say 'I know that you are scared about the shot. I will hold your hand and what you can do is close your eyes and take some big, deep breaths. It will be over quickly'.

Conversations about negative emotions represent an important learning opportunity for children. Although children may shy away from discussions of negative emotions [Denham, 1998; Laible & Panfile, 2009; Thompson, 2006], young children who are securely attached to their mothers and whose mothers also validate their emotions, are more likely to talk about negative personal experiences [Waters et al., 2010]. When parents talk to children about negative feelings, these conversations tend to be richer in emotion language and discussions of causes and consequences of emotions [Lagattuta & Wellman, 2002; Laible & Panfile, 2009; Thompson, 2006]; discussions of causes and consequences of emotions contribute to children's growing understanding of emotions. In contrast, parents can exhibit punishing contingencies in relation to their children's emotions, in essence dismissing the emotion as not important or as something that is forbidden. So, when the child fears an injection, the parent might say 'You're not really scared. Don't be a baby'. As a result, children of punishing or dismissing parents may miss out on opportunities to learn about emotional experience and to gain skills in overall emotional competence [Dadds, Sanders, Morrison & Rebetz, 1992; Gottman et al., 1997].

Whether or not parents are aware of it, children are constantly watching them as indicators of how they should respond to emotion-eliciting events. Thus, parents are both direct and indirect socializers of emotions as children frequently model their parents' patterns of behavior. For example, as measured by direct observations, preschoolers whose parents more often showed negative emotions during stressful interactions also reacted less prosocially during negative peer interactions [Dadds et al., 1992; Saarni, 1990]. In contrast, children who experience consistently positive parental emotions exhibit more prosocial tendencies during stressful, negative peer interactions [Saarni, 1990]. Observational studies also reveal that sympathetic parents, parents who accept their children's emotions and help children understand their emotions, tend to have children who cope better with stressful peer situations and who show more empathy toward their peers [Zahn-Waxler & Robinson, 1995]. On the other hand, negative or punitive reactions to children's emotions increase children's negative responses to stressful events and lead children to hide their emotions [Gottman et al., 1997]. This is detrimental to the development of emotional competence as children lose the opportunity to learn how to recognize and regulate their emotions [Casey & Fuller, 1994; Gottman et al., 1997].

Emotional Competence in the Peer Context

As we have seen, secure attachment relationships and aspects of parental socialization of emotion support young children's growing abilities to recognize their own and others' emotions, understand the causes of emotions, and employ strategies to regulate their own emotions. If children have experienced sensitive and responsive caregiving in the context of an orderly, predictable environment, children enter the world of peers at preschool age with a set of competencies that help them meet these new challenges and opportunities. In contrast, children whose family lives have been characterized by stress, instability and/or multiple sources of negative arousal enter the world of peers with fewer resources and greater vulnerability.

A growing body of research has demonstrated that aspects of emotional competence are related to positive peer relations and behavioral adjustment in preschool and kindergarten children [e.g., Denham et al., 2003; Garner & Estep, 2001]. Emotional competence helps children respond appropriately and prosocially to their peers. In turn, positive peer relationships provide a context for further refining emotional and social skills. For example, children's emotion recognition accuracy and understanding of emotions (emotion knowledge) has been shown in a meta-analysis to be positively related to social competence and negatively related to internalizing and externalizing problem behaviors, all with small to medium effect sizes [Trentacosta & Fine, 2010]. Children who recognize emotions accurately are in a position to respond appropriately and prosocially to peers. For example, recognizing that a friend is sad may prompt comforting behaviors, but misperceiving the friend's expression as angry may lead to behaviors that are less appropriate such as withdrawal or aggression. Anger perception biases have been shown to predict aggression longitudinally [e.g., Fine, Trentacosta, Izard, Mostow & Campbell, 2004]. On the other hand, preschoolers' accurate perception of anger has been linked to lower rates of being victimized by peers [Garner & Lemerise, 2007]. Thus, emotion knowledge helps children navigate the world of peers more successfully.

Children's capacity to regulate their emotions also has relevance to the peer arena. Although emotion regulation (ER) develops from infancy through adolescence and young adulthood, the preschool years are a time of rapid development of ER and the broader skills of self-regulation: 'The ability to monitor and manage one's thinking, attention, feelings, and behavior to accomplish goals' [Thompson, 2009, p. 33]. Infants and young children have limited ability to regulate their emotions, in part, because the brain areas subserving inhibitory (or effortful) control (being able to inhibit a dominant response in favor of a subdominant response) are immature [Blair, 2002; Thompson, 2009]. During their preschool years, children also gain increasing knowledge about the need to control the expression of emotion in various contexts [i.e., display rules, Saarni, 1979]. In a longitudinal study of anger expression and regulation [Cole et al., 2011], children were observed with their mothers during an 8-min wait for a gift. At 18–24 months, children quickly expressed anger and focused on the gift, and the duration of their self-initiated distraction was brief. With increasing age, children's latency to express anger and focus on the gift increased; children were quicker to initiate distraction; the duration of their distraction episodes increased, and the duration of their focus on the gift decreased [see also Supplee, Skuban, Trentacosta, Shaw & Stoltz, 2011].

Emotion regulation and the broader domain of self-regulation are considered important features of social and cognitive competence particularly critical for school readiness [Blair, 2002]. That is, with increased inhibitory control, instead of quickly reacting with negativity to frustration, children can respond more constructively to peers, wait their turn, and control their impulses in the classroom. Indeed, preschoolers higher in inhibitory control (assessed with a peg tapping task) have stronger emotion knowledge (measured with the Kusche Emotion Inventory) and greater social skills (teacher ratings) [Rhoades, Greenberg & Domitrovich, 2009]. Moreover, preschoolers' level of inhibitory control negatively correlates with teacher ratings of internalizing problem behaviors [Rhoades et al., 2009], and it predicts individual differences in conscience development [Kochanska & Aksan, 2006; Kochanska, Barry, Jimenez, Hollatz & Woodard, 2009]. Emotion regulation measured in early childhood has also been linked with decreased risk for peer rejection in middle childhood [Trentacosta & Shaw, 2009] and with decreased risk for externalizing behavior problems in middle childhood [Blandon, Calkins, Grimm, Keane & O'Brien, 2010] and adolescence [Trentacosta & Shaw, 2009].

Together, emotion understanding and emotion regulation contribute to children's emerging abilities to cope with the challenges and opportunities of the world of peers. Skill at reading others' emotions and understanding the causes and consequences of emotions helps children to understand their classmates' behavior and to respond appropriately and prosocially. More specifically, using a coping strategy to modulate emotional arousal enables children to engage in the SIP that contributes to a more socially competent response [Lemerise & Arsenio, 2000]. Being able to modulate one's fears and anxieties about approaching a group of peers also allows children to initiate the SIP that will facilitate effective choices for peer group entry (as opposed to avoiding the situation or blundering into the play and disrupting it). In some cases, emotional competence also helps children avoid peers who are volatile and aggressive, thus protecting them from victimization [e.g., Garner & Lemerise, 2007]. Children who successfully negotiate challenging peer situations have more opportunities to develop closer and more positive relationships with peers compared to children who are less successful [Ladd, 1999; Saarni, 1999]. These peer interactions and friendships are contexts in which children can further refine their emotional and social competencies.

Challenges and Opportunities for the Development of Emotional Competence: Temperament and Early Experiences

Some children face greater challenges to developing emotion regulation and self-regulation due to individual differences in aspects of temperament. Children who are high in fearful or irritable (angry) reactivity have more to regulate than do children who are lower in reactivity [Rothbart & Sheese, 2007; Thompson, 2009]. These higher levels of arousal may overwhelm children's early (and primitive) strategies for regulation. For example, children who are high in fearful reactivity may find the peer context too arousing and overwhelming, so they withdraw from peer contact. Avoiding peer contact may reduce arousal, but, at the same time, it limits the opportunity to learn coping strategies and social skills and to make friends [Rubin, Coplan & Bowker, 2009]. High levels of fearful arousal may, in fact, interfere with learning emotion regulation strategies [Blair, 2002]. On the other hand, children with high levels of angry (irritable) reactivity may respond impulsively and angrily to frustrations in peer situations, making peers wary of them. These negative behaviors may cause more socially skilled children to avoid contact with them, further depriving irritable and impulsive children of opportunities to learn social skills and to make friends [Calkins & Keane, 2009]. Children with high levels of both kinds of reactivity require more help and support from caregivers in the regulation of their emotions. Fortunately, sensitive and responsive caregiving has been shown help children develop emotion regulation skills, and caregiving is particularly important to those with greater temperamental challenges [Blair, 2002; Thompson & Meyer, 2007; see also Hastings, Kahle and Han, this vol.].

A further challenge to developing emotion regulation strategies consists of rearing environments that are high in stress and instability due to family discord and/or socioeconomic disadvantage. High levels of stress and family negative emotional climate overwhelm young children's capacities to regulate strong emotions. Thus, children whose families experience socioeconomic disadvantage and/or high levels of family stress perform more poorly on measures of regulation [e.g., Blair, 2002; Calkins & Hill, 2007; Kishiyama, Boyce, Jimenez, Perry & Knight, 2009; Lengua, Honorado & Bush, 2007] and are at risk for socioemotional adjustment problems and school failure [Blair, 2002].

For these reasons, Head Start programs have been the focus of a number of preventive interventions designed to address these risks for socioemotional problems and school failure [e.g., Bierman et al., 2008; Domitrovich, Cortes & Greenberg, 2007; Izard et al., 2008; Raver et al., 2011,

2009; Webster-Stratton, Reid & Stoolmiller, 2008]. These different programs share a focus on promoting emotional competence via curriculum components designed to improve children's emotion knowledge and emotion regulation. In addition, teachers are trained in proactive measures to support children's developing regulatory abilities by creating an orderly, predictable environment [see Webster-Stratton, 2000; Webster-Stratton et al., 2008]. These interventions have achieved success in improving children's emotion knowledge and emotion regulation as well as other indices of kindergarten readiness [e.g., Raver et al., 2011; Webster-Stratton et al., 2008]. The modifiability of emotional competence via appropriate parenting [see Webster-Stratton, 1998, for an intervention aimed at parents] and preventive interventions in preschool suggests that universal prevention programs aimed at preschoolers would be effective and associated with long term advantages in socio-emotional functioning and school adjustment. Preventive intervention during the preschool period is also important to facilitate successful transitions to kindergarten and elementary school [Rimm-Kaufman, Pianta & Cox, 2000].

Conclusions

In this chapter, we have reviewed several theories guiding research investigating how emotional competence develops in infants and young children. Whether the theory is biologically, socially, or contextually oriented, all theories emphasize the importance of accurately perceiving and identifying emotions, regulating emotions, and enacting appropriate emotional responses in emotionally charged situations. Thus, our definition of emotional competence incorporates children's abilities to use each of these key skills successfully. At the same time, successful skill development for very young children is highly dependent upon the parent-child relationship. Parenting characterized with high levels of warmth, responsiveness, and reciprocity creates the most optimal environment for successful development of emotional competence. The skills that comprise emotional competence are also crucial for successful peer relationships and have been linked to positive peer relations, behavioral adjustment, and school readiness in the preschool and early elementary school years. For children who experience challenges to developing emotional competence due to highly irritable or fearful temperament, a negatively charged family emotional climate, and/or the family stresses associated with poverty, evidence shows that warm and responsive parenting, preventive interventions aimed at parents, and universal prevention programs in preschools all can promote the development of emotional competence and behavioral adjustment. Thus, preschool is an optimal time to work with both parents and teachers to keep the development of young children's emotional competence on track as well as to improve the skills of those who may have fallen behind.

References

Bierman, K.L., Domitrovich, C.E., Nix, R.L., Gest, S.D., Welsh, J.A., Greenberg, M.T., Blair, C., Nelson, K.E., & Gill, S. (2008). Promoting academic and social-emotional school readiness: The Head Start REDI program. *Child Development, 79,* 1802–1817.

Blair, C. (2002). School readiness: Integrating cognition and emotion in a neurobiological conceptualization of children's functioning at school entry. *American Psychologist, 57,* 111–127.

Blandon, A.Y., Calkins, S.D., Grimm, K.J., Keane, S.P., & O'Brien, M. (2010). Testing a developmental cascade model of emotional and social competence and early peer acceptance. *Development & Psychopathology, 22,* 737–748.

Bretherton, I., & Munholland, K. (1999). International working models in attachment relationships: A construct revisited. In J. Cassidy & P. Shaver (Eds.), *Handbook of attachment* (pp. 89–111). New York: Guilford.

Calkins, S.D., & Hill, A. (2007). Caregiver influences on emerging emotion regulation: Biological and environmental transactions in early development. In J. Gross (Ed.), *Handbook of emotion regulation* (pp. 228–248). New York: Guilford.

Calkins, S.D., & Keane, S.P. (2009). Developmental origins of early antisocial behavior. *Development & Psychopathology, 21*, 1095–1109.

Casey, R.J., & Fuller, L. (1994). Maternal regulation of children's emotions. *Journal of Nonverbal Behavior, 18*, 57–89.

Cole, P.M., Tan, P.Z., Hall, S.E., Zhang, Y., Crnic, K.A., Blair, C.B., & Li, R. (2011). Development changes in anger expression and attention focus: Learning to wait. *Development & Psychopathology, 47*, 1078–1089.

Crick, N., & Dodge, K.A. (1994). A review of social information processing mechanisms in children's social adjustment. *Psychological Bulletin, 115*, 74–101.

Dadds, M.R., Sanders, M.R., Morrison, M., & Rebetz, M. (1992). Childhood depression and conduct disorder: An analysis of family interaction patterns in the home. *Journal of Abnormal Psychology, 101*, 505–513.

Denham, S.A. (1998). *Emotional development in young children.* New York: Guilford.

Denham, S.D., Blair, K.A., DeMulder, E., Levitas, J., Sawyer, K., Auerbach-Major, S., & Queenan, P. (2003). Preschool emotional competence: Pathway to social competence? *Child Development, 74*, 238–256.

Denham, S.D., Renwick-DeBardi, S., & Hewes, S. (1994). Emotional communication between mothers and preschoolers: Relations with social-emotional competence. *Merrill-Palmer Quarterly, 40*, 488–508.

Domitrovich, C.E., Cortes, R.C., & Greenberg, M.T. (2007). Improving young children's social and emotional competence: A randomized trial of the preschool 'PATHS' curriculum. *Journal of Primary Prevention, 28*, 67–91.

Fine, S.E., Trentacosta, C.J., Izard, C.E., Mostow, A.J., & Campbell, J.L. (2004). Anger perception, caregivers' use of physical discipline and aggression in children at risk. *Social Development, 13*, 213–228.

Garner, P.W., & Estep, K.M. (2001). Emotional competence, emotion socialization, and young children's peer-related social competence. *Early Education & Development, 12*, 29–48.

Garner, P.W., & Lemerise, E.A. (2007). The roles of behavioral adjustment and conceptions of peers and emotions in preschool children's peer victimization. *Development & Psychopathology, 19*, 57–71.

Gottman, J.M., Katz, L.F., & Hooven, C. (1997). *Meta-emotion: How familes communicate emotionally.* Mahwah: Erlbaum.

Halberstadt, A.G., Denham, S.A., & Dunsmore, J.C. (2001). Affective social competence. *Social Development, 10*, 79–119.

Izard, C.E., King, K.A., Trentacosta, C.J., Morgan, J.K., Laurenceau, J.-P., Krauthamer-Ewing, S., & Finlon, K.J. (2008). Accelerating the development of emotion competence in Head Start children: Effects on adaptive and maladaptive behavior. *Development & Psychopathology, 20*, 369–397.

Kishiyama, M.M., Boyce, W.T., Jimenez, A.M., Perry, L.M., & Knight, R.T. (2009). Socioeconomic disparities affect prefrontal function in children. *Journal of Cognitive Neuroscience, 21*, 1106–1115.

Kochanska, G. (1995). Children's temperament, mother's discipline, and security of attachment: Multiple pathways to emerging internalization. *Child Development, 66*, 597–615.

Kochanska, G. (2002). Committed compliance, moral self, and internalization: A mediated model. *Developmental Psychology, 38*, 339–351.

Kochanska, G., & Aksan, N. (2006). Children's conscience and self regulation. *Journal of Personality, 74*, 1589–1617.

Kochanska, G., Barry, R.A., Jimenez, N.B., Hollatz, A.L., & Woodard, J. (2009). Guilt and effortful control: Two mechanisms that prevent disruptive developmental trajectories. *Journal of Personality & Social Psychology, 97*, 322–333.

Kochanska, G., & Murray, K.T. (2000). Mother-child mutually responsive orientation and conscience development: From toddler to early school age. *Child Development, 71*, 417–431.

Ladd, G.W. (1999). Peer relationships and social competence during early and middle childhood. *Annual Review of Psychology, 50*, 333–359.

Lagattuta, K.H., & Wellman, H.M. (2002). Differences in early parent-child conversations about negative versus positive emotions: Implications for the development of psychological understanding. *Developmental Psychology, 38*, 564–580.

Laible, D., & Panfile, T. (2009). Mother-child reminiscing in the context of secure attachment relationships: Lessons in understanding and coping with negative emotions. In J. Quas & R. Fivush (Eds.), *Stress and memory development: Biological, social and emotional considerations* (pp. 166–195). New York: Oxford University Press.

Laible, D., & Thompson, R.A. (2000). Mother-child discourse, attachment security, shared positive affect, and early conscience development. *Child Development, 71*, 1424–1440.

Lemerise, E.A., & Arsenio, W.F. (2000). An integrated model of emotion processes and cognition in social information processing. *Child Development, 71*, 107–118.

Lengua, L.J., Honorado, E., & Bush, N.R. (2007). Contextual risk and parenting as predictors of effortful control and social competence in preschool children. *Journal of Applied Developmental Psychology, 28*, 40–55.

Mayer, J.D., & Salovey, P. (1997). What is emotional intelligence? In P. Salovey & D. Sluyter (Eds.), *Emotional development and emotional intelligence* (pp. 3–31). New York: Basic Books.

Mayer, J.D., Salovey, P., & Caruso, D.R. (2000). Models of emotional intelligence. In R.J. Sternberg (Ed.), *Handbook of human intelligence* (pp. 396–492). New York: Cambridge.

Mayer, J.D., Salovey, P., & Caruso, D.R. (2004). Emotional intelligence: Theory, findings, and implications. *Psychological Inquiry, 60*, 197–215.

Mayer, J.D., Salovey, P., Caruso, D.R., & Sitarenios, G. (2001). Emotional intelligence as a standard intelligence. *Emotion, 1*, 232–242.

Raver, C.C., Jones, S.M., Li-Grining, C.P., Zhai, F., Bub, K., & Pressler, E. (2011). CSRP's impact on low-income preschoolers' pre-academic skills: Self-regulation as a mediating mechanism. *Child Development, 82*, 362–378.

Raver, C.C., Jones, S.M., Li-Grining, C.P., Zhai, F., Metzger, M., & Solomon, B. (2009). Targeting children's behavior problems in preschool classrooms: A cluster-randomized controlled trial. *Journal of Consulting & Clinical Psychology, 77*, 302–316.

Rhoades, B.L., Greenberg, M.T., & Domitrovich, C.E. (2009). The contribution of inhibitory control to preschoolers' social-emotional competence. *Journal of Applied Psychology, 30*, 310–320.

Rimm-Kaufman, S.E., Pianta, R.C., & Cox, M.J. (2000). Teachers' judgments of the problems in the transition to kindergarten. *Early Childhood Research Quarterly, 15*, 147–166.

Rothbart, M.K., & Sheese, B.E. (2007). Temperament and emotion regulation. In J.J. Gross (Ed.), *Handbook of emotion regulation* (pp. 331–350). New York: Guilford.

Rubin, K.H., Coplan, R.J., & Bowker, J.C. (2009). Social withdrawal in childhood. *Annual Review of Psychology, 60*, 141–171.

Saarni, C. (1979). Children's understanding of display rules for expressive behavior. *Developmental Psychology, 15*, 424–429.

Saarni, C. (1990). Emotional competence: How emotions and relationships become integrated. In R.A. Thompson (Ed.), *Nebraska symposium on motivation. Vol. 36* (pp. 115–182). Lincoln: University of Nebraska Press.

Saarni, C. (1997). Coping with aversive feelings. *Motivation & Emotion, 21*, 45–63.

Saarni, C. (1999). *The development of emotional competence*. New York: Guilford.

Saarni, C., Mumme, D.L., & Campos, J. (1998). Emotional development: Action, communication, and understanding. In N. Eisenberg (Ed.), *Handbook of child psychology (5th ed.): Vol. 3. Social, emotional, and personality development* (pp. 237–309). New York: Wiley.

Supplee, L.H., Skuban, E.M., Trentacosta, C.J., Shaw, D.S., & Stoltz, E. (2011). Preschool boys' development of emotional self-regulation strategies in a sample at-risk for behavior problems. *Journal of Genetic Psychology, 172*, 95–120.

Thompson, R.A. (1998). The development of the person: Social understanding, relationships, self, conscience. In N. Eisenberg (Ed.), *Handbook of child psychology (5th ed.): Vol. 3. Social, emotional, and personality development* (pp. 24–98). New York: Wiley.

Thompson, R.A. (2006). Conversation and developing understanding: Introduction to the special issue. *Merrill-Palmer Quarterly, 52*, 1–16.

Thompson, R.A. (2009). Doing what *doesn't* come naturally: The development of self-regulation. *Zero to Three, November*, 33–39.

Thompson, R.A., & Meyer, S. (2007). The socialization of emotion regulation in the family. In J. Gross (Ed.), *Handbook of emotion regulation* (pp. 249–268). New York: Guilford.

Trentacosta, C.J., & Fine, S.E. (2010). Emotion knowledge, social competence, and behavior problems: A meta-analytic review. *Social Development, 19*, 1–29.

Trentacosta, C.J., & Shaw, D.S. (2009). Emotional self-regulation, peer rejection, and antisocial behavior: Developmental associations from early childhood to early adolescence. *Journal of Applied Developmental Psychology, 30*, 356–365. doi: 10.1016/j.appdev.2008.12.016.

Waters, E., Kondo-Ikemura, K., Posada, G., & Richters, J. (1991). Learning to love: Mechanisms and milestones. In M. Gunnar & L. Sroufe (Eds.), *Self processes and development. Minnesota symposia on child psychology* (pp. 217–255). Hillsdale: Erlbaum.

Waters, S.F., Virmani, E.B., Thompson, R.A., Meyer, S., Raikes, A., & Jochem, R. (2010). Emotion regulation and attachment: Unpacking two constructions and their association. *Journal of Psychopathology & Behavioral Assessment, 32*, 37–47.

Webster-Stratton, C. (1998). Preventing conduct problems in Head Start children: Strengthening parenting competencies. *Journal of Consulting & Clinical Psychology, 66*, 715–730.

Webster-Stratton, C. (2000). How to promote social and academic competence in young children. London: Sage.

Webster-Stratton, C., Reid, M.J., & Stoolmiller, M. (2008). Preventing conduct problems and improving school readiness: Evaluation of the Incredible Years teacher and child training programs in high-risk schools. *Journal of Child Psychology & Psychiatry, 49*, 471–488.

Zahn-Waxler, C., & Robinson, J. (1995). Empathy and guilt: Early origins of feelings of responsibility. In J. Tangney & K. Fischer (Eds.), *Self-conscious emotions* (pp. 143–173). New York: Guilford.

Elizabeth A. Lemerise
Department of Psychology, Western Kentucky University
1906 College Heights Blvd. #21030
Bowling Green, KY 42101-1030 (USA)
E-Mail Elizabeth.Lemerise@wku.edu

Hansen Lagattuta K (ed): Children and Emotion. New Insights into Developmental Affective Sciences.
Contrib Hum Dev. Basel, Karger, 2014, vol 26, pp 67–80 (DOI: 10.1159/000354355)

Emotion Socialization in the Family with an Emphasis on Culture

Linda A. Camras · Michael M. Shuster · Brittney R. Fraumeni

DePaul University, Chicago, Ill., USA

Abstract

Cultural differences in emotion responding have been widely observed and must be incorporated into any comprehensive theory of human emotion. Socialization within the family is an important conduit through which culture influences the development of emotion. In this chapter, we focus particularly on the central role that parents play in the socialization of emotion across cultures. We begin with a brief and selective historical review of theory and research on culture and emotion. We then present a highly-regarded model of parental socialization of emotion developed by Eisenberg, Cumberland and Spinrad [1998] based primarily on studies of parents and children in Western societies. Using this model as a framework, we will review the literature on cultural influences on the socialization process including parents' beliefs, goals, attitudes and values related to children's emotions and parental behaviors that may result in cultural differences in children's emotions. We then consider the emerging literature on acculturation and emotion; that is, how parental attitudes and behaviors related to emotion socialization may be modified after migration to a different cultural environment. We conclude by discussing how future studies can build upon current thinking and past research.

Our emotional lives lie at the intersection of biology and culture. This statement constitutes a point of broad agreement among contemporary scholars who may otherwise engage in vigorous and often contentious debates about the biological nature of emotion itself [Barrett, 2006 but see Izard, 2007]. Cultural differences in various aspects of the emotion process have been so widely observed that no reputable scholar can fail to recognize their import. Furthermore, to acknowledge the role of culture in emotion is to acknowledge the role of socialization in emotional development. That is, if emotion rests upon universal biological underpinnings (whatever those may be), then cultural differences must be produced via processes that take place during the course of infants', children's, and even adults' development. Reflecting the bulk of research on this topic, in this chapter, we focus on emotion socialization within the family, especially the central role that parents play in their children's emotional development. We start with a brief historical background on cross-cultural research on emotion expression.

Biology, Culture and Emotional Facial Expression

The consensus regarding the dual influences of biology and culture on emotion rests in part upon the resolution of an apparent paradox observed regarding emotional expression by scholars working in the 20th century. Numerous cultural variations in facial expression (e.g., smiling vs. crying at funerals) were documented by anthropologists throughout the 20th century [e.g., Klineberg, 1938; LaBarre, 1947]. Nevertheless, in the late 1960s, Ekman, Izard and their colleagues found that persons from a wide variety of cultures were able to recognize a set of 'prototypic' facial expressions [based on descriptions by Darwin, 1872/1998 and Tomkins, 1962] in a similar manner [e.g., Ekman & Friesen, 1971; Ekman, Sorenson & Friesen, 1969]. These findings led Ekman to conclude that recognition of emotional expression is universal across cultures, a conclusion that has since become widely accepted [but see Russell, 1994].

To resolve the apparent conflict between the findings of his recognition research and the views of anthropologists, Ekman [1972] developed his 'neurocultural theory of emotion.' This theory proposed a species-universal set of innate emotions and corresponding emotional facial expressions. However, over the course of development, infants, children and even adults may learn to modify their emotional expressivity in accordance with the standards and norms of their culture. Such cultural 'display rules' may mandate one who experiences an emotion to minimize, amplify, or completely hide the expression of that emotion or even to mask it with the display of a different emotion. More recently, researchers have also demonstrated differences in the finer morphological details of emotional expression prototypes produced by members of different cultures, a notion captured by the concept of emotional expression 'dialects' [Elfenbein & Ambady, 2003].

Emotion Socialization

Within the realm of developmental psychology, Ekman's research initially led to a wave of studies on children's recognition of emotional expression [e.g., Field & Walden, 1982; Odom & Lemond, 1972]. However, more recently, researchers have also turned their attention to the role of culture in the development of other aspects of children's emotions, including the process of emotion socialization. Because this research rests on models based on studies of American children, we begin with a brief discussion of emotion socialization as it is treated in the Western literature.

Perhaps the most influential model of emotion socialization was presented over a decade ago by Eisenberg, Cumberland and Spinrad [1998]. Focusing on the role of parents, these scholars designated four categories of emotion-related socialization behaviors: (a) parents' own emotional expression; (b) their reactions to the child's emotions (i.e., contingent responding); (c) discussion of emotion with or in the presence of the child, and (d) parents' selection of potential emotion-inducing situations that children encounter (i.e., via 'niche picking'). Importantly, emotion socializing behaviors may be produced with or without parents' explicit intention to influence their children's behaviors and emotions. Furthermore, several categories of emotion-related socialization behaviors may occur in a single episode.

Eisenberg et al.'s [1998] model identifies a number of factors that influence parents' emotion socializing behaviors. These include cultural factors (i.e., cultural beliefs, norms, and values related to emotion), but also parents' personal beliefs, values, goals, and attitudes that may be consistent or inconsistent with those of the larger society. In addition, Eisenberg et al. [1998] acknowledge other relevant influences including child characteristics (e.g., age, temperament), parent characteristics (e.g., personality, gender), and contextual factors (e.g., the public vs. private nature of an emotion episode). Central to the topic of this chapter, one important feature of the model (and indeed much developmental research on emotion socialization) is a focus on child behavioral outcomes that are judged more (or less) desirable in terms of their cultural appropriateness and social desirability.

For Western cultures, such child behaviors are thought to reflect a balance between seeking personal goals and maintaining good relationships with others. This notion is captured in the concept of social 'competence' [Eisenberg et al., 1998; Rubin, Bukowski & Parker, 2006]. Emotion competence is thought to contribute to social competence in that it allows children to regulate their behavior in a socially competent manner. Although the component skills proposed to underlie emotion competence have varied [e.g., Halberstadt, Denham & Dunsmore, 2001; Saarni, 1999], most scholars recognize that they include children's ability to understand their own and others' emotions as well as their ability to manifest their own emotions in a socially and culturally appropriate manner.

While most research on emotion socialization has focused on children from Western backgrounds, Eisenberg et al.'s [1998] model can readily be applied as a framework for reviewing the smaller body of research that has been conducted on emotion socialization in non-Western cultures as well as research that has drawn comparisons across cultures. We begin our review, however, with one aspect of the model that is not typically considered in studies that are restricted to European and North American children – parents' beliefs, values, goals, and attitudes regarding children and emotion.

Parental Beliefs, Values, Goals, and Attitudes about Children and Emotion

Although cultures may differ on a number of dimensions [Hofstede, 1980] most current research on children and emotion focuses on differences between collectivistic and individualistic cultures. Collectivistic cultures encourage interdependence among ingroup members and consequently value emotions reflecting a person in relation to the group. In contrast, individualistic cultures encourage personal independence and value emotions that are expressions of individuality [Markus & Kitayama, 1991].

These values may be reflected in emotion socialization goals. For instance, in a survey study conducted with European-American mothers and Chinese mothers, nearly half of the European-American mothers thought it was necessary for their children to develop a sense of emotional honesty and to be able to process their feelings, whereas no Chinese mothers thought this was important [Chao, 1995]. Interestingly, different cultural values may underlie some similarities in parents' emotion-related goals for their children in different cultures. For example, Cheah and Rubin [2003] found that American and Chinese mothers both consider controlling negative emotions important for children, but for different reasons. American mothers thought it was a beneficial practice for the child's own development whereas Chinese mothers thought it was important because it enabled children to adhere to social conventions. Similarities in emotion socialization can also arise from different beliefs about development. For example, Kelley and Tseng [1992] found that American and Chinese parents thought emotion socialization was important for 6- to 8-year-old children but again it was for different reasons. American mothers thought that children of this age had begun to develop a clearer sense of self whereas Chinese mothers thought children had begun to develop a better sense of their place in society.

In a questionnaire study that included 48 different nations, Diener & Lucas [2004] asked college students about their desires for their children's emotions (i.e., happiness, fearlessness, and anger suppression). They found that respondents from all countries desired happiness for their children but those from individualistic nations targeted higher levels of happiness than did those from collectivistic cultures. For the remaining two emotions (fearlessness and anger suppression), the biggest difference was found between genders rather than cultures; participants wanted their sons to be more fearless and engage in more anger suppression than their daughters.

While collectivism and individualism are important cultural dimensions, emotion socialization may also be influenced by other features of culture. Halberstadt & Lozada [2011] discussed three other factors that might potentially influence emotion socialization: power-distance, children's place in the family, and the ways children learn. Power-distance distinguishes societies in terms of vertical or horizontal orientations of power. Vertical societies emphasize more power distinctions and value obedience to authority figures while horizontal societies affirm greater equality. Children's place in the family refers to the value placed on children in the society and the reasons behind their value. For instance, some cultures see children as an economic benefit whereas others see them as psychologically beneficial. Regarding the way children learn, Halberstadt and Lozada [2011] identified four key elements related to children's emotional development: 'when,' 'whether,' 'who,' and 'how'. Different cultures have different beliefs about *when* their children are capable of learning to perceive and appropriately express emotions. Cultures also differ in parents' beliefs about *whether* children develop through maturation or direct teaching. Among cultures that assume learning happens through direct teaching, there may be differences in *who* is thought to be in charge of teaching (e.g., parents or other children). There also are many different beliefs in *how* children learn, including how they learn about emotion: discipline, telling, active participation, scaffolding, and discussion. For example, immigrant Chinese-American mothers believe 'training' and discipline are needed, whereas European-American mothers utilize more discussion [Chao, 1994, 1995].

In an innovative empirical study using a focus-group methodology [Parker et al., 2012], moderators led discussions about emotion with mothers from three different sub-cultures within the United States: European-American, African-American, and Lumbee-American Indians. Within these discussions, a number of themes emerged, including some that had not been theoretically predicted by the investigators. Both cultural similarities and differences were found. For example, cultural similarities included an emphasis on emotional connections with children, emotion contagion within the family, and intergenerational change in emotion socialization. Cultural differences were found in beliefs about children's emotional privacy and the importance of discussion in emotion socialization. Specifically, Lumbee-American-Indian groups thought it was important to always know what their children were feeling, whereas European-American groups thought it was critical that their children keep their emotions to themselves for a while to reflect on what they were feeling before they shared.

Research conducted on parental beliefs, values, goals, and attitudes about emotion rests on the dual assumptions that these reflect the values of the parents' culture (at least in part) and that they influence parents' actual socialization behaviors. Relatively few studies have directly examined these relationships by measuring cultural and/or parental values and parental behaviors in the same investigation. However, in one study, Rao, McHale and Pearson [2003] found that valuing children's socioemotional development was associated with self-reported use of authoritative parenting practices among both Chinese and Indian mothers.

Parent Emotional Expressivity

Eisenberg et al.'s [1998] model proposes that parents' own expression of emotion is an important component of emotion socialization. Parents' emotional expression can result in elicitation of corresponding emotions in the child (e.g., mutual positive affect) and/or similar tendencies to be more or less expressive in general. At the same time, parental expression does not always result in correspondence between parent and child. For example, parental anger expression may elicit fear and anxiety in children and/or result in the suppression of children's emotional expressivity [Camras & Shuster, 2013; Eisenberg et al., 1998].

Cultures considered to be individualistic generally endorse emotional expressivity more than cultures considered to be collectivistic. However, this generalization must be qualified by consideration of the particular emotion being expressed and the particular context in which expression takes place [Matsumoto et al., 2008; Mesquita & Leu, 2007]. In general, positive emotions as well as negative emotions related to self-assertion (e.g., anger, contempt, disgust) are more acceptable in individualistic cultures such as the U.S. and Canada [Safdar et al., 2009]. In contrast, expression of negative emotions that reflect or promote interdependence (e.g., sadness, shame) may be considered more desirable in collectivistic cultures such as Japan or China [Miller, Fung, Lin, Chen & Boldt, 2012; Matsumoto et al., 2008].

Investigations of parental emotional expressivity are sometimes – but not always – consistent with the general trends described above. For example, Camras, Kolmodin and Chen [2008] found that European-American mothers reported expressing more positive emotion than did Mainland Chinese mothers using the Self-Expressiveness in the Family Questionnaire (SEFQ), a measure that queries parents about a wide range of situations in which emotion may (or may not) be expressed. In one of the few cultural comparisons that assessed parental emotional expressivity using observational measures, Wörmann, Holodynski, Kärtner and Keller [2012] found that German mothers smiled more when interacting with their 4-month-old infants than did African mothers from the Nso culture in Cameroon. However, in contrast, Kisilevsky et al. [1998] observed no differences in smiling by Chinese and Canadian mothers during face-to-face interactions with 3- to 6-month-old infants. The differing results for these two observational studies (both of which compared an individualistic to a collectivistic culture) highlight the importance of considering other potentially important factors influencing parental emotional expressivity (e.g., beliefs about infants' receptivity to emotional expression).

Regarding negative emotions, in the context of socializing proper behavior, Chinese parents have been found to express more anger-related feelings (e.g., disapproval, criticism) than do European-American parents [Camras, Sun, Li & Wright, 2012; Fung, 1999; Wu et al., 2002]. This stands in contrast to the general trend for self-assertive negative emotions (such as anger) to be expressed less often in collectivist cultures than in individualistic cultures. Paradoxically, Chinese parents' expression of such self-assertive negative emotion is designed to induce shame (an interdependence-related negative emotion) in their children. This example highlights the importance of considering the interplay among multiple factors (e.g., cultural values, socialization goals, power relationships) to understand parents' emotion-related socialization behavior in specific situational contexts.

Other studies comparing different collectivistic or different individualistic cultures suggest a similar conclusion. For example, Zevalkink and Riksen-Walraven [2001] observed Japanese mothers to express more positive regard than both Indonesian and Dutch mothers when interacting with their children in a structured play session. Their study is particularly noteworthy in that it demonstrated differences between two collectivist cultures (Japan and Indonesia) and also greater positive expressivity in one collectivistic culture (Japan) than in an individualistic culture (The Netherlands). The authors suggest that socioeconomic differences between their Japanese sample and the other two groups might be responsible for the observed differences in maternal positive expressivity. Regarding negative emotion, Camras, Kolmodin & Chen [2008] failed to find a difference between Mainland Chinese and European-American mothers in their self-reported overall display of negative emotions on the SEFQ. However, self-assertive versus interdependence-related emotions (e.g., anger vs. shame) were grouped together in their study. Possibly, cultural differences would have been found if these had been examined separately.

Studies in Western cultures generally have found that parents' positive expressivity is related to greater socioemotional adjustment in children although findings for negative emotional expressivity have been inconsistent [Halberstadt & Eaton, 2003]. Relations between parental expressivity and child adjustment have not generally been studied in other cultures. However, in one investigation of Indonesian children [Eisenberg, Liew & Pidada, 2001], some unexpected findings were obtained. Parental positive expressivity was unrelated to children's social functioning. In contrast, greater negative expressivity was associated with poorer social functioning, possibly due to its effects on children's emotion regulation. These findings highlight the need for further investigations of relationships between parental expressivity and children's social and emotional competence and adjustment across cultures.

Parents' Contingent Responding to Children's Emotions

Most studies of parental emotion socialization focus on contingent responding to children's behavior and/or expression of emotion. Like parents' own expression of emotion, contingent responding provides children with information about what types of emotion and emotional expression are appropriate. Parent responses can serve to reinforce or punish the child's emotional behavior or can present the child with a model of a more appropriate response [Camras & Shuster, 2013; Eisenberg et al., 1998]. Parents' own expression of emotion often occurs in the context of their responses to their children's emotional displays.

Cultural differences have been found in several studies that have examined parental contingent responding to children. Generally, these differences have been plausibly explained in terms of what is known or believed about cultural values and corresponding parental socialization goals. For example, Cole and Tamang [1998] found that Brahmin and Tamang mothers in Nepal reported different types of responding to children's anger directed toward the mother. Brahmin mothers said that they would most often instruct the child regarding how to behave while Tamang mothers reported that they would 'try to make the child happy' by cajoling or acceding to the child's demand (e.g., for more food at a meal). The researchers interpreted these findings as being consistent with Brahmins' greater acceptance and expectation of anger and their emphasis on parents' responsibility to teach children to control their anger rather than avoid anger altogether. In contrast, Tamang mothers believed that experiencing anger should be avoided but that children will learn this by themselves. The researchers also speculated that Brahmins' self-perceived higher social status (i.e., greater power) was a factor underlying their greater acceptance of anger as an appropriate emotion even within this collectivistic culture.

In a subsequent observational study, Cole, Tamang and Shrestha [2006] found that Tamang adults often respond to children's anger by teasing; for example, by accompanying their reprimands with humor rather than showing anger themselves. As in Cole's previous study, Brahmin adults instructed children more than Tamang adults but they also more often cajoled or acceded to children's demands (again, often for food). Curiously, this latter finding contradicts the self-reports that Brahmin and Tamang mothers' provided in the preceding study. Such apparent contradictions are possibly attributable to differences in the types of anger situations being considered in the two studies [i.e., mother-directed anger in Cole & Tamang, 1998 and both adult- and peer-directed anger in Cole, Tamang & Shrestha, 2006]. Alternatively, they may exemplify the possibility that self-reports sometimes reflect parental intentions and goals more than their actual behaviors when confronted with a real-life situation.

Nonetheless, self-report studies continue to provide valuable information regarding parent socialization of emotion, especially when data is collected from both parents and children. For example, Raval and Martini [2009] found that mothers' self-reported beliefs and behaviors were related to their 5- to 9-year-old children's self-reported emotional responses in a study that compared Gujarati Indian mothers living in the old city versus a more modern suburb. Raval and Martini's study also highlighted differences in adherence to traditional values and behaviors that may exist among members of the same culture. Old-city mothers believed that children's expressions of anger and sadness were less acceptable than did the more modern suburban mothers. Correspondingly, old city mothers reported that they punished these emotions more. Raval and Martini's [2009] study illustrates again that overly broad generalizations regarding emotion-related differences between collectivist versus individualist cultures may prove untenable. For example, their finding regarding old city mothers' disapproval of children's sadness displays appears to contradict conclusions reached by Safdar et al. [2009] regarding greater acceptance of sadness within collectivist cultures. Differences between the two studies may be due to differences in the age of the expressers being considered (children vs. adults) or the contexts in which sadness is presumed to be displayed (e.g., whether or not sadness is seen to promote collectivistic goals of interdependence or relatedness within the particular context).

Rarely considered is the interesting possibility that the same parental contingent response might have somewhat different effects on children from different cultures. Such results were obtained recently by Trommsdorff and Friedlmeier [2010] in an observational study of Japanese versus German mothers' contingent responses to their preschooler daughters' distress. Within both cultures, mothers' sensitivity to their child's distress was positively related to their daughter's greater sympathy toward others. However, within the context of the child-distress episode itself, German and Japanese mothers' sensitivity were related to different child responses. Greater sensitivity by German mothers was related to their daughter's maintaining distress for a longer period of time while greater sensitivity by Japanese mothers was related to more rapid lessening of their daughter's distress. To explain these differences, the researchers proposed that within the context of a culture that promotes independence, German mothers' sensitivity served to encourage their daughters' greater expression of self-focused emotion.

As indicated earlier, research on emotion socialization in European-American families often focuses on developing children's social and emotional competence (i.e., encouraging child behaviors that are judged to be socially appropriate). Much of this research involves the study of Western parents' contingent responding to children's emotions using Richard Fabes' Coping with Children's Negative Emotions measure (CCNES)

[Fabes, Poulin, Eisenberg & Madden-Derdich, 2002]. The CCNES is a self-report measure in which parents indicate how they would respond to their children's expressions of negative emotion in a variety of situations (e.g., having to perform in public, being unable to attend a party due to illness). Results have suggested that disparaging or punishing a child's undesirable emotion is less effective in encouraging socially appropriate responding than is 'emotion coaching' (i.e., encouraging the child's expression of emotion and helping him or her develop strategies for more effective coping with the eliciting situation and their own emotional response). For example, Kennedy Root and Stifter [2010] found that maternal emotion coaching benefited temperamentally exuberant children's preschool adjustment. Fabes, Poulin, Eisenberg and Madden-Derdich [2002] found that positive emotion coaching was related to better emotion recognition skills in preschool children. Correspondingly, European-American mothers reported using the more effective strategies most often.

A few studies have investigated mothers' contingent responses to children's emotions in non-Western cultures using modified versions of the CCNES. Because these studies have not included Western participants, conclusions regarding cultural similarities and differences have been inferred based on inspecting patterns in the data. For example, Friedlmeier, Corapci and Cole [2011] construe these patterns as suggesting that parents in at least some non-Western cultures (e.g., China, India) tend to actively discourage emotional expression more than do European-American parents. However, variability also occurs among mothers within any particular culture. For example, Chan, Bowes and Wyver [2009] found differences among Hong Kong mothers in the extent to which they valued relational emotion competence goals (i.e., promoting interpersonal harmony) and individualistic emotion competence goals (i.e., promoting children's self-esteem). Mothers with more individualist goals tended to encourage their children's expression of emotion and use emotion coaching strategies, while mothers with more relational goals were more likely to dismiss their children's expressions of negative emotion (primarily distress). Since these researchers did not directly examine children's social or emotional competence, no conclusions can be made regarding relations between mothers' goals and behaviors and children's emotional development.

In fact, few studies have directly examined relationships between mothers' emotion socialization goals or behaviors and children's competence and adjustment in non-Western cultures. This is particularly surprising since an implicit assumption in the literature seems to be that culturally normative emotion socialization behaviors would result in emotion competence (i.e., culturally appropriate emotion responding) which in turn would be related to positive social emotional adjustment. As described above, Raval and Martini [2009] did find that maternal discouragement of emotional expression was related to children's self-reported expression regulation (presumably a culturally-competent form of behavior); however, they did not consider relations between maternal emotion socialization and other indices of social emotional adjustment (e.g., internalizing or externalizing behaviors). Interestingly, the few studies that have examined such relationships have found both similarities and differences between findings reported in studies of Western and non-Western children. For example, Tao, Zhou and Wang [2010] found that maternal punishment responses to children's negative emotion predicted poorer parent-, teacher- and child-rated adjustment while emotion-focused and problem-focused coping responses predicted better adjustment in Hong Kong children (as they do for European-American children). However, in contrast to US findings, maternal minimization of emotion was not related to poorer adjustment, and maternal encouragement of emotional expression was not related to better adjustment.

Similar findings for minimization and expression encouragement have been reported for Turkish children [Friedlmeier et al., 2011]. Friedlmeier et al. [2011] suggest that maternal minimization responses may be interpreted differently by children from different cultures and thus may have different effects. For example, children may be more accepting of parental pressure to regulate their expressivity if they perceive such regulation to be culturally normative. Consequently, parental minimization may not negatively impact their social emotional adjustment.

Discussion of Emotion

In a seminal observational study of British families, Dunn and Brown [1994] found that family discussion of emotion was related to greater emotion understanding in 2- to 4-year-old children. Because emotion understanding is considered an important component of social and emotional competence, a number of subsequent studies have investigated parents' emotion-related speech to infants and children in both Western and non-Western cultures [see also Fivush, this vol.; Hughes et al., this vol.].

Even in infancy, cultural differences have been found in mothers' verbalizations during interactions with their babies. For example, Bornstein et al. [1992] found that Japanese mothers used more affectionate speech during free-play interactions with their 13-month-old infants than did US and French mothers. This difference might plausibly be related to Japanese mothers' goals of creating a close relationship of interdependence between mother and child as opposed to American mothers' goal of fostering infants' independence via focusing their attention on the outside world [Rothbaum, Pott, Azuma, Miyake & Weisz, 2000]. Interestingly, the amount of Japanese mothers' affectionate speech also exceeded that of Argentine mothers, again highlighting the existence of differences among collectivist cultures. Furthermore, given the very limited language capabilities of 13-month-olds, it is worth noting that the mechanism underlying any socialization effects of affectionate speech on infants probably would involve the positive prosodic and facial expressivity that presumably would accompany the mothers' verbal statements.

Several investigators have studied emotion-related talk in Chinese and European-American families in preschool and school-age children. For example, Miller et al. [2012] conducted a highly detailed study of narrative practices in Taiwanese and European-American families. While conversational stories about children's past experiences were common in both cultures, the Taiwanese families used these stories as a framework for socializing proper behavior in their children while American parents used them to affirm the child's preferences and strengths and to encourage their self-esteem. Thus, as indicated earlier, the Taiwanese parents focused on misconduct and shame more than American parents while American parents tended to use humor even when recounting children's misdeeds.

When talking specifically about emotion, Chinese mothers have been found to provide fewer explanations regarding causal antecedents than European-American mothers [Wang, 2001]. This difference in maternal behavior might provide a plausible explanation for findings regarding Chinese children's lesser knowledge regarding emotion situations [Wang, 2003; Wang, Hutt, Kulkofsky, McDermott & Wei, 2006]. More recently, Doan and Wang [2010] confirmed this predicted relationship in a study that explicitly examined associations between maternal discussion and child emotion knowledge in European-American and immigrant Chinese children. Chinese mothers were again found to talk less about emotion than European-American mothers and individual differences in children's emotion understanding positively correlated with maternal discussion of people's thoughts and feelings in both European-American and Chinese immigrant families.

Immigration and Emotion Socialization

Doan and Wang's [2010] investigation is one of a small number of studies that have looked at families undergoing cultural change (i.e., immigrant families moving from one culture to another). Overall, research shows that the emotion-socializing attitudes and behaviors of immigrant parents fall somewhere in between those characterizing their culture of origin and their culture of destination. For example, Camras et al. [2008] found that European-American mothers reported showing more positive expressivity than mothers from mainland China and that Chinese immigrant mothers fell in between the two other groups. Ispa et al. [2004] reported that levels of maternal warmth (as manifested in verbal expressions of love, attentiveness, and admiration) by Mexican-American immigrants increased as acculturation increased and mothers moved toward the parenting style of the new culture. Cervantes [2002] showed that Mexican immigrant mothers used more emotion explanations than emotion labels when talking to their preschool children while more acculturated Mexican-American mothers provided similar amounts of labels and explanations.

Parental behavior observed among immigrant families reflects the influence of both *acculturation* [i.e., shifting ones' values, attitudes and behaviors toward those of the new culture, Burnam, Telles, Karno, Hough & Escobar, 1987] and *enculturation* [i.e., retaining one's original cultural heritage, Davidson & Cardemil, 2009]. For example, Perez-Rivera and Dunsmore [2011] studied 40 mothers who emigrated from various parts of Latin America to the United States. Mothers' higher Latino enculturation predicted a stronger belief in guiding their children's emotions. In addition, mothers with higher Anglo acculturation were less likely to believe that children's emotions can be dangerous. Thus, Latino-American immigrants' emotion socializing strategies and goals incorporated components from both their old and new cultures.

Researchers stress that disparities in parent-child acculturation levels have notable consequences for emotional relationships between parents and children. For example, Qin [2006] proposed that as the cross-generational acculturation gap increases, so does the emotional distance between parents and their children. Therefore, parents who fall far behind their children's level of acculturation may become less influential emotion socialization agents. Related to this, Tardif and Geva [2006] found that high acculturation disparity between Chinese immigrant parents and their 13- to 15-year-old children was associated with reports of a greater number of conflicts regarding interpersonal issues (although not with the emotional intensity of these conflicts). Conversely, mothers and adolescents in the low acculturation disparity group reported more conflict regarding chores and other daily activities. More work is needed to examine how the combination of traditional and new emotion socialization practices influences child outcomes.

Research on acculturation and emotion in adults may also provide important insight into the influence of parental cultural change on emotion socialization. Theorists suggest that emotion patterns acculturate due to the changing requirements of the new environment and may cause immigrants to appraise the same situation differently. For example, De Leersnyder, Mesquita and Kim [2011] found that the similarity between the emotional responses of Turkish immigrants to Belgium and native citizens of Belgium depended on the amount of time the immigrants had spent in Belgium and the number of their social contacts with people of this new culture.

Conclusions and Future Directions

In our increasingly global society, a greater understanding of the role of culture in human development has become paramount. Parenting is an important conduit through which culture influences children's socialization experiences and consequently their development. In recent decades, developmentalists' thinking about this process has become more sophisticated and a number of conceptually-oriented articles and chapters have been published that have informed and guided the structure our current review [primarily Eisenberg et al., 1998 but also Bornstein & Lansford, 2010; Cole & Tan, 2007; Dunsmore & Halberstadt, 2009; Halberstadt & Lozada, 2011]. Virtually all of these appear to share the basic assumption that culture influences parenting beliefs, values, goals and attitudes, which themselves influence parenting behaviors, which in turn influence children's outcomes. Our review of the research generally upholds this consensual view. At the same time, we have pointed to several aspects of the process that deserve further empirical consideration. We close with some general statements that may suggest how future studies can build upon current thinking and past research.

There Is More to Culture than Individualism/ Collectivism

While consideration of this cultural dimension has led to important advances in our understanding of parenting and development, it is not the only factor that distinguishes among cultures. In his seminal research, Hofstede [1980] identified a number of additional cultural dimensions (e.g., uncertainty avoidance) that may be equally or even more important in terms of guiding parental goals, values, attitudes, and behaviors. Other scholars also have identified further cultural beliefs and values that may impact parenting practices [see especially Halberstadt & Lozada, 2011]. Thus, future research should attend to a wider range of cultural factors that may impact children's emotion socialization.

Mothers are Not the Only Agents of Emotion Socialization

For practical reasons, most investigations of emotion socialization within the family have examined only mothers [see Fivush, this vol.; Hughes et al., this vol.]. Yet, one study that compared respondents in 48 different countries found that males and females often have different emotion goals for their children [Diener & Lucas, 2004]. Although recruiting fathers to participate in research may be challenging, greater effort should be made to do so. It is also likely that siblings (especially older siblings) play an important role in emotion socialization. Thus siblings' own emotional expressions, contingent responding to the target child's emotion, and emotion-related discussion also merit systematic study.

Post Hoc Explanations Deserve Follow-Up Investigation

Although a large number of studies have demonstrated cultural differences in children's emotional responding or emotion understanding, we excluded several of them from this review because they did not involve direct measures of parent socialization [e.g., Tenenbaum, Visscher, Pons & Harris, 2004; Markham & Wang, 1996]. Frequently, these studies interpret their findings in terms of cultural beliefs, attitudes, values, or goals that presumably influence parental behavior. These studies constitute important first steps in the research process. There is a strong need, however, to replicate these original results and to test the proposed explanations directly by assessing cultural values, parental behaviors, and children's outcomes in the same investigation.

Mind the Gap (between Word and Deed)

Due to their greater feasibility, most studies of emotion socialization across cultures have involved questionnaire and interview data rather than direct observations of socialization behaviors. While assuming that parents are accurate reporters of their own actions may seem logical, caution dictates that further attention be directed to empirical examination of the relationships between self-report and observational data gathered in various situational contexts within different cultures. Thus, more observational studies need to be conducted. Furthermore, when observational studies involve an interpretative component (e.g., identifying instances of 'positive affect'), then indigenous culture members should participate in the development and implementation of the behavioral coding system.

Final Thoughts

Contemporary scholars appear to have arrived at a consensual view of emotion socialization that acknowledges cultural influences on parenting beliefs, values, goals and attitudes which themselves influence parenting behaviors which in turn influence children's social emotional behaviors and adjustment. Examining the entire process in a single investigation constitutes the next challenge. Although such studies may require larger sample sizes than have been utilized in previous investigations, recent developments across the globe make such large-scale studies more feasible. For example, growing research communities in non-Western nations offer greater possibilities for developing cross-cultural collaborative relationships that will enable the collection of larger data sets. Such collaborative relationships also can facilitate the development of more relevant and valid assessments of culture and socialization based on the insights of non-Western researchers. In addition, the spread of the internet and various online technologies have made long-distance collaborations both practical and convenient. Importantly, such collaborations could potentially involve sharing video recordings of parenting behaviors and family interactions as well as collecting questionnaire data. These possibilities encourage us to look forward to a new generation of research on culture, emotion socialization within the family, and children's development.

References

Barrett, L.F. (2006). Are emotions natural kinds? *Perspectives on Psychological Science, 1*, 28–58.

Bornstein, M.H., & Lansford, J. (2010). Parenting in M.H. Bornstein (Ed.), *Handbook of cultural developmental science,* (pp. 259–277). NY: Psychology Press.

Bornstein, M.H., Tal, J., Rahn, C., Galperin, C.Z., Pêcheux, M.G., Lamour, M., Toda, S., Azuma, H., Ogino, M., & Tamis-LeMonda, C.S. (1992). Functional analysis of the contents of maternal speech to infants of 5 and 13 months in four cultures: Argentina, France, Japan, and the United States. *Developmental Psychology, 28*, 593–601.

Burnam, M.A., Telles, C.A., Karno, M., Hough, R.L., & Escobar, J.I. (1987). Measurement of acculturation in a community population of Mexican Americans. *Hispanic Journal of Behavioral Sciences, 9*, 105–130.

Camras, L.A., Kolmodin, K., & Chen, Y. (2008). Mothers' self-reported emotional expression in Mainland Chinese, Chinese American and European American families. *International Journal of Behavioral Development, 32*, 459–463.

Camras, L.A., & Shuster, M. (2013). Current emotion research in developmental psychology. *Emotion Review*, 321–329.

Camras, L.A., Sun, K., Li, Y., & Wright, M.F. (2012). Do Chinese and American children's interpretations of parenting moderate links between perceived parenting and child adjustment? *Parenting, 12*, 306–327.

Cervantes, C.A. (2002). Explanatory emotion talk in Mexican immigrant and Mexican American families. *Hispanic Journal of Behavioral Sciences, 24*, 138–163.

Chan, S.M., Bowes, J., & Wyver, S. (2009). Parenting style as a context for emotion socialization. *Early Education and Development, 20*, 631–656.

Chao, R.K. (1994). Beyond parental control and authoritarian parenting style: Understanding Chinese parenting through the cultural notion of training. *Child Development, 65*, 1111–1119.

Chao, R.K. (1995). Chinese and European American cultural models of the self reflected in mothers' childrearing beliefs. *Ethos, 23*, 328–354.

Cheah, C.S.L., & Rubin, K.H. (2003). European American and mainland Chinese mothers' socialization beliefs regarding preschoolers' social skills. *Parenting: Science and Practice, 3*, 1–21.

Cole, P.M., & Tamang, B.L. (1998). Nepali children's ideas about emotional displays in hypothetical challenges. *Developmental Psychology, 34*, 640–646.

Cole, P., Tamang, B., & Shrestha, S. (2006). Cultural variations in the socialization of young children's anger and shame. *Child Development, 77*, 1137–1151.

Cole, P.M., & Tan, P.Z. (2007). Emotion socialization from a cultural perspective. In J.E. Grusec, & P.D., Hastings (Eds.), *Handbook of Socialization: Theory and Research*, (pp. 516–542). NY: Guilford Press.

Davidson, T.M., & Cardemil, E.V. (2009). Parent-child communication and parental involvement in Latino adolescents. *Journal of Early Adolescence, 29*, 99–121.

Darwin, C. (1998). *The expression of the emotions in man and animals*. New York: Oxford University Press. (Original work published 1872.)

De Leersnyder, J., Mesquita, B., & Kim, H.S. (2011). Where do my emotions belong? A study of immigrants' emotional acculturation. *Personality and Social Psychology Bulletin, 37*, 451–463.

Diener, M.L., & Lucas, R.E. (2004). Adults' desires for children's emotions across 48 countries: Associations with individual and national characteristics. *Journal of Cross-Cultural Psychology, 35*, 525–547.

Doan, S.N., & Wang, Q. (2010). Maternal discussions of mental states and behaviors: Relations to emotion situation knowledge in European American and immigrant Chinese children. *Child Development, 81*, 1490–1503.

Dunn, J., & Brown, J. (1994). Affect expression in the family, children's understanding of emotions, and their interactions with others. *Merrill-Palmer Quarterly: Journal of Developmental Psychology, 1982*, 120–137.

Dunsmore, J.C., & Halberstadt, A.G. (2009). The dynamic cultural context of emotion socialization. In J.A. Mancini & K.A. Roberto (Eds.), *Pathways of human development: Explorations of change* (pp. 171–190). Lanham: Lexington Books/Rowman & Littlefield.

Eisenberg, N., Cumberland, A., & Spinrad, T.L. (1998). Parental socialization of emotion. *Psychological Inquiry, 9*, 241–273.

Eisenberg, N., Liew, J., & Pidada, S.U. (2001). The relations of parental emotional expressivity with quality of Indonesian children's social functioning. *Emotion, 1*, 116–136.

Ekman, P. (1972). Universals and cultural differences in facial expressions of emotion. In J. Cole (Ed.), *Nebraska Symposium on Motivation: Vol. 19. Current Theory and Research in Motivation* (pp. 207–283). Lincoln: University of Nebraska Press.

Ekman, P., & Friesen, W.V. (1971). Constants across cultures in the face and emotion. *Journal of Personality and Social Psychology, 17*, 124–129.

Ekman, P., Sorenson, E., & Friesen, W. (1969). Pan-cultural elements in facial display of emotion. *Science, 164*, 86–88.

Elfenbein, H.A., & Ambady, N. (2003). Universals and cultural differences in recognizing emotions. *Current Directions in Psychological Science, 12*, 159–164.

Fabes, R.A., Poulin, R.E., Eisenberg, N., & Madden-Derdich, D.A. (2002). The coping with children's negative emotions scale (CCNES): Psychometric properties and relations with children's emotional competence. *Marriage & Family Review, 34*, 285–310.

Field, T.M., & Walden, T.A. (1982). Production and discrimination of facial expressions by preschool children. *Child Development, 53*, 1299–1311.

Friedlmeier, W., Corapci, F., & Cole, P.M. (2011). Emotion socialization in cross-cultural perspective. *Social and Personality Psychology Compass, 5*, 410–427.

Fung, H. (1999). Becoming a moral child: The socialization of shame among young Chinese children. *Ethos, 27*, 180–209.

Halberstadt, A.G., & Eaton, K. (2003). A meta-analysis of family expressiveness and children's emotion expressiveness and understanding. *Marriage and Family Review, 34*, 35–62.

Halberstadt, A.G., Denham, S.A., & Dunsmore, J.C. (2001). Affective social competence. *Social Development, 10*, 79–119.

Halberstadt, A.G., & Lozada, F.T. (2011). Emotion development in infancy through the lens of culture. *Emotion Review, 3*, 158–168.

Hofstede, G. (1980). *Culture's consequences: International differences in work-related values*. Sage Publications, Incorporated.

Ispa, J.M., Fine, M.A., Halgunseth, L.C., Harper, S., Robinson, J.A., Boyce, L., Brooks-Gunn, J., & Brady-Smith, C. (2004). Maternal intrusiveness, maternal warmth, and mother-toddler relationship outcomes: Variations across low-income ethnic and acculturation groups. *Child Development, 75*, 1613–1631.

Izard, C.E. (2007). Basic emotions, natural kinds, emotion schemas, and a new paradigm. *Perspectives on Psychological Science, 2*, 260–280.

Kelley, M.L., & Tseng, H.M. (1992). Cultural differences in child rearing: A comparison of immigrant Chinese and Caucasian American mothers. *Journal of Cross-Cultural Psychology, 23*, 444–455.

Kennedy Root, A. & Stifter, C. (2010). Temperament and maternal emotion socialization beliefs as predictors of early childhood social behavior in the laboratory and classroom. *Parenting: Science and Practice, 10*, 241–257.

Kisilevsky, B.S., Hains, S.M.J., Lee, K., Muir, D.W., Xu, F., Fu, G., & Yang, R.L. (1998). The still-face effect in Chinese and Canadian 3- to 6-month-old infants. *Developmental Psychology, 34*, 629–638.

Klineberg, O. (1938). Emotional expression in Chinese literature. *Journal of Abnormal and Social Psychology, 33*, 517–520.

LaBarre, W. (1947). The cultural basis of emotions and gestures. *Journal of Personality, 16*, 49–68.

Markham, R., & Wang, L. (1996). Recognition of emotion by Chinese and Australian children. *Journal of Cross-Cultural Psychology, 27*, 616–643.

Markus, H.R., & Kitayama, S. (1991). Culture and the self: Implications for cognition, emotion, and motivation. *Psychological Review, 98*, 224–253.

Matsumoto, D., Yoo, S.H., Fontaine, J., Anguas-Wong, A.M., Arriola, M., Ataca, B., & Grossi, E. (2008). Mapping expressive differences around the world: The relationship between emotional display rules and individualism versus collectivism. *Journal of Cross-Cultural Psychology, 39*, 55–74.

Mesquita, B., & Leu, J. (2007). The cultural psychology of emotion. In S. Kitayama & D. Cohen (Eds.), *Handbook of Cultural Psychology* (pp. 734–759). New York: Guilford Press.

Miller, P., Fung, H., Lin, S., Chen, E., & Boldt, B. (2012). How socialization happens on the ground: Narrative practices as alternate socializing pathways in Taiwanese and European-American families. *Monographs of the Society for Research in Child Development, 77*, 1–125.

Odom, R.D., & Lemond, C.M. (1972). Developmental differences in the perception and production of facial expressions. *Child Development, 43*, 359–369.

Parker, A.E., Halberstadt, A.G., Dunsmore, J.C., Townley, G., Bryant, A. Jr., Thompson, J.A., & Beale, K.S. (2012). 'Emotions are a window into one's heart': A qualitative analysis of parental beliefs about children's emotions across three ethnic groups. *Monographs of the Society for Research in Child Development, 77*, 1–144.

Perez Rivera, M.B., & Dunsmore, J.C. (2011). Mothers' acculturation and beliefs about emotions, mother-child emotion discourse, and children's emotion understanding in Latino families. *Early Education and Development, 22*, 324–354.

Qin, D. (2006). 'Our child doesn't talk to us anymore': Alienation in immigrant Chinese families. *Anthropology & Education Quarterly, 37*, 162–179.

Rao, N., McHale, J.P., & Pearson, E. (2003). Links between socialization goals and child-rearing practices in Chinese and Indian mothers. *Infant and Child Development, 12*, 475–492.

Raval, V.V., & Martini, T.S. (2009). Maternal socialization of children's anger, sadness, and physical pain in two communities in Gujarat, India. *International Journal of Behavioral Development, 33*, 215–229.

Rothbaum, F., Pott, M., Azuma, H., Miyake, K., & Weisz, J. (2000). The development of close relationships in Japan and the United States: Paths of symbiotic harmony and generative tension. *Child Development, 71*, 1121–1142.

Rubin, K.H., Bukowski, W.M., & Parker, J.G. (2006). Peer interactions, relationships, and groups. In N. Eisenberg, W. Damon & R.M. Lerner (Eds.), *Handbook of Child Psychology: Vol. 3, Social, Emotional, and Personality Development* (6th ed., pp. 571–645). Hoboken, NJ: John Wiley & Sons Inc.

Russell, J.A. (1994). Is there universal recognition of emotion from facial expression?: A review of the cross-cultural studies. *Psychological Bulletin, 115*, 102–141.

Saarni, C. (1999). *The Development of Emotional Competence.* New York: Guilford Press.

Safdar, S., Friedlmeier, W., Matsumoto, D., Yoo, S.H., Kwantes, C.T., Kakai, H., & Shigemasu, E. (2009). Variations of emotional display rules within and across cultures: A comparison between Canada, USA, and Japan. *Canadian Journal of Behavioural Science/Revue canadienne des sciences du comportement, 41*, 1–10.

Tao, A., Zhou, Q., & Wang, Y. (2010). Parental reactions to children's negative emotions: Prospective relations to Chinese children's psychological adjustment. *Journal of Family Psychology, 24*, 135–144.

Tardif, C.Y., & Geva, E. (2006). The link between acculturation disparity and conflict among Chinese Canadian immigrant mother-adolescent dyads. *Journal of Cross-Cultural Psychology, 37*, 191–211.

Tenenbaum, H.R., Visscher, P., Pons, F., & Harris, P.L. (2004). Emotional understanding in Quechua children from an agro-pastoralist village. *International Journal of Behavioral Development, 28*, 471–478.

Tomkins, S. (1962). *Affect, Imagery, Consciousness: Vol. 1: The Positive Affects.* New York: Springer.

Trommsdorff, G., & Friedlmeier, W. (2010). Preschool girls' distress and mothers' sensitivity in Japan and Germany. *European Journal of Developmental Psychology, 7*, 350–370.

Wang, Q. (2001). 'Did you have fun?': American and Chinese mother-child conversations about shared emotional experiences. *Cognitive Development, 16*, 693–715.

Wang, Q. (2003). Emotion situation knowledge in American and Chinese preschool children and adults. *Cognition & Emotion, 17*, 725–746.

Wang, Q., Hutt, R., Kulkofsky, S., McDermott, M., & Wei, R. (2006). Emotion situation knowledge and autobiographical memory in Chinese, immigrant Chinese, and European American 3-year-olds. *Journal of Cognition and Development, 7*, 95–118.

Wörmann, V., Holodynski, M., Kärtner, J., & Keller, H. (2012). A cross-cultural comparison of the development of the social smile: A longitudinal study of maternal and infant imitation in 6- and 12-week-old infants. *Infant Behavior and Development, 35*, 335–347.

Wu, P., Robinson, C.C., Yang, C., Hart, C.H., Olsen, S.F., Porter, C.L., & Wu, X. (2002). Similarities and differences in mothers' parenting of preschoolers in China and the United States. *International Journal of Behavioral Development, 26*, 481–491.

Zevalkink, J., & Riksen-Walraven, J.M. (2001). Parenting in Indonesia: Inter- and intracultural differences in mothers' interactions with their young children. *International Journal of Behavioral Development, 25*, 167–175.

Linda A. Camras, PhD
Department of Psychology, DePaul University
2219 N. Kenmore Ave.
Chicago, IL-60659 (USA)
E-Mail lcamras@depaul.edu

Hansen Lagattuta K (ed): Children and Emotion. New Insights into Developmental Affective Sciences.
Contrib Hum Dev. Basel, Karger, 2014, vol 26, pp 81–94 (DOI: 10.1159/000354360)

Gender and Voice in Emotional Reminiscing

Robyn Fivush
Department of Psychology, Emory University, Atlanta, Ga., USA

Abstract
Using sociocultural and feminist theories as frames, I argue that parentally guided reminiscing about past emotional experiences is a critical site for the socialization of children's developing emotional voice. Moreover, this process is gendered. Research on parent-child reminiscing about the emotional past indicates that mothers are more elaborative and emotionally expressive than fathers, and, overall, both mothers and fathers are more elaborative and emotionally expressive when reminiscing about the emotional past with their preschool daughters as compared to sons. These early gender differences are reflected in children's and adolescents' personal narratives about emotional experiences, with girls telling more elaborated and emotionally expressive narratives than boys across development. Importantly, these gender differences are specific to personal narratives; both boys and girls narrate stories about their parents' childhood experiences in ways consistent with the parents' gender, not their own. Both parental reminiscing style and adolescents' personal and intergenerational narratives are related to emotional well-being, although there are some suggestions that these relations are gendered as well. The overall patterns suggest that children are developing an emotional voice that reflects their understanding of their emotional lives.

When we talk about the past, we talk about emotions. We share our experiences in everyday conversations, over the phone, over the internet and over the dinner table, and in these sharings we talk not just about what happened but how we and others felt about it, why it was important, exciting, embarrassing, upsetting, fun. In fact, much of everyday conversation is filled with stories we share about our experiences, whether of our day or our life. Studies of spontaneous conversations indicate that narrative sharing of our past occurs approximately every 5 min [Bohanek, Fivush, Zaman, Lepore, Merchant & Duke, 2009], and individuals indicate that they share more than 90% of their daily emotional experiences with another in conversation within 48 h of its occurrence [Rime, 2007].

In this chapter, I explore both the forms and the functions of emotional reminiscing, why this is such a critical site for the socialization of emotion, and how constructing coherent, emotionally expressive narratives about past experiences helps children and adolescents to both understand and regulate their emotional selves. Using sociocultural and feminist theoretical frames, I argue that children are creating an emotional 'voice' through socioculturally structured narrative interactions, in the sense that individuals develop a specific way of narrating their emotional experiences that reflect their understanding of their emotional life. Moreover, these voices are gendered, such that girls are learning to be more emotionally expressive and to understand themselves as emotional beings to a greater extent than are boys beginning early in the preschool years and continuing through adolescence.

Sociocultural Approaches to Emotion

Vygotsky [1978] argued that all social and cognitive skills begin on the interpersonal plane, between people, and are then internalized into the intrapersonal plane, as an individual skill. Cultures provide both the functions and the tools for skills deemed necessary to be a competent member of that culture. At the most global level, the culture provides a set of shared values and scripts for understanding and enacting cultural norms. These culturally shared values are learned at the local level, in structured interactions in which more competent members of the culture both model and mold the performance of less competent cultural members. Through these local social interactions, individuals learn both the forms and values of behaving and believing certain ways of being in the world.

From this perspective, emotions are conceptualized as interpersonal constructs as much as intrapersonal constructs [see also Fischer & Manstead, 2008; Lazarus, 2006; Saarni, 2008]. The ways in which emotions are culturally understood will be communicated through parentally structured activities that help inform the developing child the appropriate ways to label, experience, and express emotion. This argument is similar to other theoretical arguments in the literature that emotions are part of culturally mediated scripts that modulate how emotions are experienced and expressed, and are embedded within culturally mediated norms of behavior [e.g., Saarni, 2008; Widen & Russell, 2008]. Importantly, from a Vygotskian perspective, language is the consummate cultural tool through which these understandings are communicated [Fivush & Nelson, 2004]. Through language, children gain access to explicit shared understandings of activities. Language allows for a more structured, sequenced and nuanced shared set of cultural values and forms. Thus, the ways in which emotions are talked about is critical for children's developing emotional understanding. Certainly, how emotions are discussed in the moment is important, and chapters throughout this volume [Camras et al., Hughes et al., Lemerise et al.] demonstrate the critical role of parental socialization of ongoing emotion through language [see also Eisenberg, Spinrad & Eggum, 2010, for a theoretical discussion]. Here, I focus on how parentally structured narratives about *past* emotional experiences are a critical site for the socialization of emotion, and more specifically, of an emotional voice.

Why Narratives Are Critical

When experiencing 'hot' emotions, emotions in the moment, the child (and parent) must cope with the immediate environment, from the physiological arousal, to the behavioral expression, to the environmental conditions in which the emotion is embedded. A good example is a toddler's temper tantrum in a supermarket. Every parent and, indeed every adult within hearing range, knows how difficult it is to reason with a child in this context. The goal is usually simply to control the child's emotional outburst and get out of the store! In contrast, when sitting down later that day to discuss what happened, the parent and child are in a much different situation. Now parent and child can reflect on what happened, what caused the child's behavior, how and why the child expressed their emotion in the way they did, what might have been better strategies for expressing or regulating that emotions, and the consequences of these different forms of expression [see Dunn, Brown & Beardsall, 1991; Harris, 2008, for related arguments]. This discussion takes the form of a narrative, essentially a story about what happened.

Narratives are the process and the product of how humans understand their experiences [McAdams, 2001; McLean, Pasupathi & Pals, 2007]. Narratives provide a canonical linguistic structure for organizing events into beginnings, middles, and ends [Bruner, 1990; Fivush & Nelson, 2004], providing a coherent chronological sequence of what happened. But narratives move beyond simple chronologies. Narratives include what Bruner [1990] has called the landscape of consciousness, integrating information about thoughts and emotions, why things happened the way they did, how the self and others thought and felt about that, and how these thoughts and emotions led to particular consequences over others. In essence, narratives provide a seamless integration of the inner and outer worlds to provide a coherent account of human experiences, replete with understanding how inner states cause and are caused by external occurrences. In this way, narratives provide linguistic guides to how to understand one's emotional experiences. Stemming from Vygotskian theory, parents help structure these more coherent narratives in ways that help their children understand their own experiences in particularly culturally mediated ways.

Voice and Silence

The use of narrative reconstruction to express, elaborate and explain emotional experiences in particular ways resonates with feminist ideas about *voice* and *silence*. Although there are many varieties of feminist theory [Rosser & Miller, 2000], all converge on several key assumptions about knowledge. First, knowledge is always contexted; individuals perceive the world from a particular social, historical, and cultural place. In this sense, feminist theories are similar to sociocultural theory that postulates that all knowledge is mediated through cultural lenses. Objectivity is possible, but only through the concatenation of multiple subjective perspectives [Bordo, 1990]. Second, knowledge is constructed in local social situations in which particular perspectives are highlighted or foregrounded. Again, this is similar to sociocultural theory that postulates that cultures emphasize particular ways of understanding the world that impart cultural skills and values. In addition, feminist theories introduce the concept of voice and silence [Belenky, Clinchy, Goldberger & Tarule, 1986; Gilligan, 1982]. Voice comes from a position of cultural power, in which one is allowed to provide their perspective on an event, and that perspective is heard and validated [Gergen, 2001]. In contrast, silence is when an individual is either not allowed to tell what happened and/or their version is dismissed or negated. At a cultural level, an example is sexual violence against women. In the historical changes since the second wave of the women's movement, the ways in which victims of sexual violence have been allowed to tell their stories has changed dramatically [Fivush, 2010].

Consideration of voice and silence allows for a more nuanced understanding of parent-child narratives about emotional experiences [Fivush, 2004]. When parents structure narratives in ways that allow their child to express their own experience, and this experience is validated, the child will come to 'own' this experience as authentic. In contrast, when the parent does not allow the child 'voice' or negates the child's experience, the child will learn not to trust their own experiential account. For emotional events, this can happen at multiple levels. At the most global level, certain kinds of emotional events may simply never be talked about. If a parent does not allow a child to talk about experiences of anger, for example, the child may learn that anger is simply an inappropriate emotion and will learn to cope with anger very differently than if the parent acknowledges anger and helps the child create a coherent explanatory narratives of these kinds of experiences that provide both validation of the emotion and regulatory strategies. At a more nuanced level, even within narratives of an emotional experience, parents can validate a specific emotional response, and/or provide an explanatory structure, and/or provide regulatory strategies. By focusing on specific aspects of emotional experience, parents may be modeling and teaching their children that different aspects of emotions are important, valid, and self-defining. Thus, it is not just *whether* something is voiced, but *how* it is voiced. As we will review, research over the past 20 years has demonstrated individual differences in how parents engage in emotional reminiscing, and that these differences are related to gender of both parent and child leading to gendered ways of understanding oneself as an emotional being [see Fivush, 2007; Fivush, Haden & Reese, 2006; Fivush & Zaman, in press, for reviews].

To provide some flesh to these arguments, here are two examples from mothers with their 4-year-old child discussing a time the child was angry [from Fivush, Brotman, Buckner & Fivush, 2000]. The first is a mother and daughter discussing an event with the child's brother:

Mother: Well, I seem to remember that yesterday you and Patrick were swinging on the swings and he was doing something that really annoyed you. Do you remember?

Child: He wouldn't give me a swing.

Mother: Oh! That's right…and did you wait patiently for a long time, hmm?

Child: Yes.

Mother: And is that when you started to get really angry? Uh-huh, how do you feel inside when you get angry?

Child: …mad.

Mother: Mad! And did your mouth turn down at the corners? And do you feel like going grrr?

In this example, the mother identifies a time the child felt angry and identifies the event with an emotion label (annoyed), thus immediately attributing a particular emotional state to the child. When the child relays what happened, the mother elaborates on this, again mentioning the child's emotional state (waiting patiently). Thus the mother provides a causal explanation for the resulting anger, and moves the conversation into a discussion of the emotional state of anger itself, both attributing anger to her daughter and providing information about how anger is expressed facially, verbally, and 'inside'. Note that the mother uses multiple emotion words, and quite sophisticated ones for a 4-year-old (annoyed, patient), and she provides a full narrative about what caused the emotion and how it felt, although there is no resolution. Contrast this with the following mother and her 4-year-old son, also discussing a time the child was angry:

Mother: Now how do you feel when Mommy makes you take your vitamins in the morning and you don't want to take them?

Child: I feel mad.

Mother: You do! And what do you do?

Child: I hide.

Mother: Uh-huh, then what happens to Mommy? How does Mommy feel when you don't take your vitamins and your calcium?

Child: Mad.

Mother: Then what happens to you?

Child: Get in trouble.

Mother: Yeah.

Here, the mother begins with the external event and asks the child to provide how he felt, rather than labeling the emotion for the child as in the first example. The mother does not dwell on any aspect of the emotional experience; in fact, she does not even use an emotion word. Rather she focuses on the consequences of the child's anger, both in terms of causing another person's emotion, and it terms of behavioral consequences for the child. In the first example, the overall narrative focuses on how and why the child felt as she did, exploring how it feels to be angry, and using multiple nuanced descriptors of the emotion. In this example, the narrative focuses on the external events rather than the emotional experience itself, there are few and nondifferentiated emotion terms used ('mad' by the child, 'feel' by the mother). Both convey a sense of story but the first voices the emotion very differently than the second.

In summary, from both sociocultural and feminist approaches, emotion understanding and regulation develops within socially structured interactions in which parents guide children into culturally appropriate ways of expressing and explaining their emotional experiences. Narratives about past emotional experiences are critical in this process because narratives allow for both a coherent explanatory framework, and because, through narrating the past, certain experiences, and especially certain aspects of experiences, are highlighted, or voiced, whereas other aspects may be silenced. Thus, from these perspectives, the ways in which parents structure narratives about the emotional past with their children is a critical site for the socialization of emotion.

Parent-Child Emotional Reminiscing

Reminiscing about the shared past emerges very early in development [see Fivush, 2007, for a review]. Virtually as soon as children begin talking they begin participating in conversations about their past experiences, although early on, these conversations are led by parents, with children participating by confirming, negating or providing just a detail or two. By age 3, most children begin to participate more in these conversations, often bringing the past up as a topic of conversation, and providing multiple answers to adult questions. By the end of the preschool years, most children are able to provide a fairly coherent narrative of a past experience. This pattern coincides with children's developing ability to talk about their emotional experiences, with 2-year-olds using a few emotion words, an increasing ability to integrate emotional language into conversational interactions across the preschool years, and the ability to describe and explain emotional experiences by the end of the preschool years [see Harris, 2008, for a review]. Importantly, for both autobiographical narratives and emotion understanding, there are large individual differences across development that are at least partly attributable to parental socialization.

Substantial research has demonstrated that parents, especially mothers, show enduring individual differences in how they structure narratives about the shared past with their preschool children, and some of this work has focused specifically on narratives of emotional experience. Two aspects of emotion narratives have been studied: level of elaboration and the emotion content. Most of the research has been conducted with broadly middle class White Western mothers, although there is more limited research with fathers and with other cultures. A full discussion of culture is beyond the scope of this chapter [but see Wang, in press; Camras et al., this vol.]. Here, I will discuss how gender of parent and child influence emotional reminiscing across development.

Elaborative Reminiscing Style

Level of elaboration refers to the extent to which the parent provides a fully detailed, rich and coherent narrative about the past event [Fivush et al., 2006]. In elaborated narratives, the parent incorporates information the child provides into the next question, including more details to create a more richly detailed and coherent story. In contrast, parents who are low in elaboration essentially ask few and redundant questions, and they rarely provide new details with each question. Although there is sparse longitudinal research on reminiscing with fathers [but see Reese, Haden, & Fivush, 1996], maternal reminiscing style is stable across development. Mothers who are highly elaborative early in the preschool years are still more highly elaborative than their low elaborative peers at the end of the preschool years [see Fivush et al., 2006, for a review]. Importantly, however, reminiscing style is not related to general talkativeness. Mothers who are highly elaborative when reminiscing are not necessarily more talkative in other contexts such as book reading, free play or care giving contexts [Haden & Fivush, 1996].

This pattern indicates that reminiscing is a special context in which mothers have implicit and/or explicit strategic goals of helping their children to understand their experiences in particular ways. Indeed, Kulkofsky, Wang and Kim Koh [2009] found that more highly elaborative mothers report using these conversations more as a tool to help their children to understand themselves and to create a shared history with their child, than do less elaborative mothers. Through creating richly detailed and coherent narratives about the past, highly elaborative mothers are helping their children to develop a more embellished personal history, and in this way, are helping their children to focus on past experiences as self-defining. In support of this interpretation, mothers who are more highly elaborative and emotionally expressive have children who show a more coherent and differentiated self-concept both concurrently and longitudinally [Bird & Reese, 2006; Wang, Doan & Song, 2010; Welch-Ross, Fasig & Farrar, 1999]. Indeed, recent research has extended this finding to adolescence, such that mothers who are more highly elaborative when reminiscing with their preschoolers longitudinally predicts to adolescent self-esteem [Reese, Yan, Jack & Hayne, 2010].

Emotional Content of Reminiscing

A second individual difference in how parents structure narratives about the emotional past with their children focuses on the emotional content of these conversations [see Fivush, 2007; Fivush & Zaman, in press, for reviews]. Emotional content has been conceptualized as the number of emotion words used, as well as the number of different emotion words used (e.g., saying 'sad' three times versus saying 'sad', 'unhappy', and 'upset'), as a marker for levels of nuance and differentiation in emotion discussions. In addition, the ways in which emotions are integrated into the narratives has been examined as attributions of emotion ('You were so sad'), causes of emotions ('You were sad because you could not play with your friend') and resolutions of emotions ('But I played with you and then you felt better'). Perhaps not surprisingly, it matters what type of emotion is being discussed. Mothers spend more time talking about the causes and resolutions of negative than positive events overall [Lagattuta & Wellman, 2002; Sales, Fivush & Peterson, 2003], and within types of negative events, mothers spend more time explaining causes and resolutions of fear than for sadness or anger, and more time resolving sadness than anger [Fivush, Berlin, Sales, Mennuti-Washburn & Cassidy, 2003]. These patterns again suggest that reminiscing about the emotional past provides a unique context for parents to help their children to understand their emotional lives in particular ways. Provocatively, these patterns are also gendered.

Gender Differences in Parent-Child Emotional Reminiscing

There are differences between mothers and fathers, and differences in the ways in which both mothers and fathers reminisce about emotional events with daughters as compared to sons. Although there is limited research on emotional reminiscing that includes fathers, all the studies converge on finding that mothers are more elaborative with their preschoolers when reminiscing about emotional events than are fathers [Reese, Haden & Fivush, 1993, 1996; Zaman & Fivush, in press; see Fivush & Zaman, in press, for a review].

In addition, mothers talk more about emotion overall, they use more emotion words and more unique emotions words than do fathers [Adams, Kuebli, Boyle & Fivush, 1995; Kuebli & Fivush, 1992; Kuebli, Butler & Fivush, 1995], and they discuss the causes of emotions with children in greater detail than fathers [Fivush et al., 2000]. These patterns continue into childhood. Both in spontaneous conversations around the dinner table [Bohanek et al., 2009] and in elicited family reminiscing about emotional events with 9- to 12-year-old children [Bohanek, Marin & Fivush, 2008; Fivush, Marin, McWilliams & Bohanek, 2009], mothers are more elaborative overall than are fathers, and mothers talk more about the causes of emotions than do fathers. These parental gender differences in emotional reminiscing provide models for young children about how to understand their own emotional experiences in gendered ways. Females are more elaborative, emotionally expressive, and explanatory than are males.

Parents also differentiate reminiscing with daughters and sons. Both mothers and fathers are more elaborative with daughters than with sons [Reese & Fivush, 1993; Reese et al., 1993], and mothers of daughters in particular are more elaborative than mothers of sons [Reese & Newcombe, 2007]. It must be noted that many studies do not find that maternal reminiscing differs as a function of child gender, but when differences are obtained, they are always in this direction. All studies that have included fathers have found that fathers are more elaborative with daughters than with sons [see Fivush & Zaman, in press, for a review]. Both mothers and fathers also talk more about emotion overall, and especially talk more about sadness, with daughters than with sons [Adams et al., 1995; Fivush et al., 2000; Kuebli & Fivush, 1992; Kuebli et al., 1995]. Mothers use a greater variety of emotion words with daughters than with sons [Kuebli & Fivush, 1992], and are more likely to provide resolutions for emotional experiences, especially sadness, with daughters than with sons [Fivush, 1989].

Finally, the themes of parent-child reminiscing differ by both gender of parent and gender of child. Mothers focus more on interpersonal and relational themes than do fathers [Buckner & Fivush, 2000; Fivush et al., 2000]. For mothers, emotions are embedded in a web of connections to others, with emotions being caused by other people (you were sad when your friend moved away) and resolved with other people (you wrote her a letter and then you felt better). For fathers, emotions are more likely to be embedded in an autonomous theme (you were sad because you lost your favorite toy), and resolutions rarely include emotional connections with others. These differences are mirrored in daughter versus son conversations, in that both mothers and fathers place emotions in a more interpersonal framework when reminiscing with daughters than with sons [Fiese & Skillman, 2000; Fivush & Buckner, 2003].

Several things must be emphasized. First, reminiscing is dyadic and likely bidirectional. Gender differences in parent-child reminiscing are a function of both parent and child. Several longitudinal and intervention studies, however, indicate that parental reminiscing early in development uniquely predicts both children's personal narratives and emotion understanding later in development [see Fivush et al., 2006, for a full review] indicating that, although certainly bidirectional, what parents do matters for outcome. Second, reminiscing is reconstructive. The argument is not that parents and children narrate accurate portrayals of the past, but that in reminiscing, certain ways of understanding the past are voiced. Girls are being exposed to emotional reminiscing that is more expressive, more differentiated, more relational, and more focused on resolutions and regulation of emotional experiences than are boys. Thus, both the gendered models provided by maternal as compared to paternal reminiscing and the differentiated way in which both mothers and fathers reminisce about emotional experiences with daughters than with sons, converge on constructing an emotional voice that is more elaborated, expressive and regulated for females than for males.

Reminiscing Style and Children's Emotional Understanding

There is substantial research demonstrating that parents (with most of the research focusing on mothers) who talk more about emotions, and talk more about how to understand and regulate emotional experiences, have children who show higher levels of emotional understanding and regulation [see Eisenberg et al., 2010; Harris, 2008; Hughes et al., this vol; Lemerise et al., this vol., for overviews]. In most of this research, no distinction is made between talk about the present and talk about the past. Based on my earlier arguments, emotional *reminiscing* should play a unique role in children's developing emotional understanding. In two studies where this was directly examined, maternal reminiscing style predicted more variance in preschool children's emotional understanding as assessed on standardized tasks than maternal emotion talk in other contexts, including free play and book reading [Laible, 2004; Reese & Cleveland, 2006]. These studies did not examine gender of child. Although there are small but robust gender differences in emotional understanding and regulation favoring girls [Brody & Hall, 2008], there is little research specifically linking gender differences in parental reminiscing style to the obtained gender differences in emotional understanding and regulation. This is an important avenue for future research.

Relations between paternal reminiscing and child outcomes have also received minimal attention. Bohanek et al. [2008] examined family narratives in families with 9- to 12-year-old children reminiscing about highly positive and negative experiences they had shared. Mothers engaged in these family narratives in more elaborated and emotionally expressive ways than did fathers. Further, mothers who engaged in more emotionally expressive and explanatory narratives had children with higher levels of emotional well-being, as assessed by maternal report of internalizing and externalizing behaviors. Surprisingly, fathers who engaged in more emotionally expressive and explanatory reminiscing had children who showed lower levels of maternally reported emotional well-being. Because we assessed parental reminiscing within the full family context, we were not able to examine gender of child effects, as most families had more than one child participating, often of different genders. Although this finding is hard to explain, it might be that fathers who go against stereotype create difficulties for their pre-adolescent children.

To complicate this further, these same families were assessed in spontaneous family reminiscing that emerged around the dinner table [Bohanek et al., 2009]. Within these typical dinnertime conversations, two types of narratives emerged: shared family stories that focused on events the family shared in the remote past, weeks or months ago, such as family vacations or outings; and 'Today I' narratives, where family members shared with each other the events of their day. Here again, in both types of narratives, mothers were more elaborative than fathers. In addition, mothers who engaged in more elaborated reminiscing about shared family past events had pre-adolescents who showed lower maternally reported internalizing and externalizing behaviors; confirming the results seen with elicited narratives. Although fathers' contributions to these shared family stories from the past were unrelated to child emotional well-being, fathers who elaborated more on narratives about the events of the day (e.g., sharing stories with their children about what had just happened at school or at band practice that day) had pre-adolescents who showed fewer internalizing and externalizing behaviors. In contrast, mothers' contributions to these 'Today I' stories were unrelated to child well-being.

So, mothers may play a more important role in developing children's emotional wellbeing by keeping alive and discussing shared family experiences from the past, whereas fathers may contribute to children's well-being by keeping up to date on daily emotional events [see Fivush, Bohanek, Marin & Duke, 2010, for a full discussion].

The Emergence of a Gendered Emotional Voice

Stemming from the theoretical perspective argued here, gendered parental reminiscing should be internalized in ways that lead to an individual voice. Indeed, girls begin to tell more emotionally expressive personal narratives early in childhood, and these differences remain consistent across development. Buckner and Fivush [1998] found that 7-year-old girls told more elaborated and emotionally expressive narratives about emotional experiences such as feeling lonely, or feeling close to another, than did boys. Girls were also more likely to place their narratives within an ongoing social relationship (feeling lonely because they had a fight with their best friend, with the narrative focusing on how upsetting the rift in the relationship is) than did boys (feeling lonely because they were not picked for a sports team, with the narrative focusing on feeling bad that they did not get to play baseball). Girls continue to tell more evaluative narratives than do boys. For example, Pasupathi and Wainryb [2010] found that across middle childhood, girls and boys did not differ in the amount of factual information provided about their personal experiences, but girl's narratives include more evaluative information than did boys. In middle adolescence, girls tell more elaborated personal narratives about both positive and negative personal experiences, and these narratives include more specific emotion ('I was sad') and more general affect ('It was a hard time in my life') [Bohanek & Fivush, 2010; Fivush et al., 2011]. These gender differences remain consistent across adulthood, with female adults telling more elaborated and emotionally expressive personal narratives than do males [Bauer, Stennes & Haight, 2003; Cross & Madson, 1997; Niedzwienska, 2003], and, as already reviewed, these differences are again mirrored in parental reminiscing, thus completing the cycle.

This cycle of more elaborated emotionally expressive narration from mother to daughter is embedded in larger family and cultural interactions in which females generally talk more than males and are generally more emotionally expressive. A cascade of cultural and developmental factors lead to females engaging in more emotional reminiscing, leading to greater practice and therefore skill at this activity. This is exactly in accord with sociocultural theories that argue that children are drawn into, and become skilled at, activities that their cultures values; here, the wrinkle is that within cultures, gender plays a critical role in how activities are structured and come to be valued across development [see Fivush & Zaman, in press, for a full theoretical discussion]. A further wrinkle is that this more elaborated emotionally expressive reminiscing may have both positive outcomes, as discussed in this chapter, but also more negative outcomes. Rumination, which can be considered an extreme form of expressive reminiscing, is a risk factor in the development of depression, and is higher among females beginning in adolescence [Nolen-Hoeksema, Wisco & Lyubomirsky, 2008]; adolescent females co-ruminate more than adolescent males both with their friends and with their mothers [Rose, Carlson & Waller, 2007]. How and when reminiscing turns to rumination is an important question for future research.

It is also critical to determine whether these gender differences reflect how individuals understand their emotional selves. One way to address this is to examine whether this reflects a more general narrative style, such that females would tell more elaborated emotionally expressive narratives about any protagonist than do males. A related question is whether children are telling these more elaborated and emotionally expressive narratives by modeling their parents' reminiscing style.

Intergenerational Narratives

We addressed these questions in a study of adolescents (13–16 years old) asked to tell both highly positive and negative personal narratives, as well as to tell stories they knew about their parents when their parents were growing up, what we labeled intergenerational narratives [see Fivush et al., 2011, for a review]. We were interested in intergenerational narratives for multiple reasons. First, these stories provide frameworks or models for adolescents to understand their place in the family, and thus to understand themselves in relation to others [Fiese & Bickham, 2004; Fivush, Bohanek & Duke, 2005; Norris, Kuiack & Pratt, 2004]. Second, in asking adolescents to tell stories about their mothers and their fathers, we could examine similarities and differences between how they told these gendered stories and how they told their own personal gendered story. Finally, we could examine how the ways in which personal and intergenerational narratives were told related to adolescents' emotional well-being. Given that females place their own experiences in a more social relational context, we reasoned that, for girls, knowing stories, especially about their mothers, might influence their personal well-being to greater extent than for boys.

Turning first to the stories that adolescents told about their parents' childhoods, both boys and girls told stories about their mothers that were more elaborated and emotionally expressive than the stories they told about their fathers [Zaman & Fivush, 2011]. Note that when these same adolescents were asked to narrate personal experiences, girls told more elaborated and emotionally expressive narratives than did boys [Fivush et al., 2011]. The intergenerational stories most likely reflect how the parents told the story to the child, but also reflect how the adolescent has heard and understood the story. Thus, both boys and girls tell stories about their mothers and their fathers that reflect the parents' gender, but stories about themselves that reflects their own gender. This indicates that boys know how to tell more elaborated and emotionally expressive narratives (and girls do not always tell more elaborated and emotionally expressive narratives), but when boys tell narrative about themselves they choose not to use this style. In fact, boys' narratives about their mothers were more emotionally expressive than their personal narratives!

We then examined whether adolescents used their parents stories as models for their own personal narratives. Thus, we compared adolescents' personal and intergenerational narratives [Merrill, Walsh, Zaman & Fivush, 2011]. Girls told stories about themselves that were similar to the stories they told about their mothers in coherence and emotionality. More specifically, girls who told more thematically coherent stories (stories that provided more elaborated links between actions) about their mothers' childhood that included more specific emotion words and general affective evaluations told personal narratives with these same characteristics. There were no relations between girls' personal narratives and the stories they told about their fathers. For boys, there were no relations at all between their personal narratives and stories they told about either their mothers or their fathers. Thus, girls seem to be using their mothers as narrative models, but boys do not seem to be using either parent as such.

Relations to Emotional Well-Being

Given that a more elaborated and emotionally expressive parental reminiscing style early in development is related to children's developing emotional understanding and regulation, as reviewed above, an interesting question is the extent to which children's developing personal narrative style is related to their emotional well-being [Bohanek & Fivush, 2010]. Boys who told personal narratives that included more expression of both specific emotion words and more general affect showed lower levels of maternally reported internalizing behaviors. There were no relations between how girls narrated their emotional past and their emotional well-being. Remember that this is in the context of girls telling more emotionally expressive narratives overall. So even though girls tell more emotionally expressive narratives than boys, there are no relations to well-being, and even though boys' generally tell less emotionally expressive narratives than girls, those boys who do tell more emotionally expressive personal narratives show higher emotional well-being.

In contrast, for the intergenerational narratives, girls who told stories about their mothers that were more emotionally expressive showed lower levels of both maternally reported internalizing and externalizing behaviors. There were no relations between girls' intergenerational stories about their fathers and their well-being. And for boys, there were no relations between intergenerational stories about either mothers or fathers and their well-being. Thus, well-being is related to more emotionally expressive personal narratives for boys, but not to intergenerational narratives, whereas well-being is related to more emotionally expressive maternal intergenerational narratives for girls, but not personal narratives. This surprising finding suggests that girls' well-being may be more interpersonally situated, with family stories playing a role in their sense of well-being, whereas boys' well-being stems from a more autonomous perspective.

Gendered Reminiscing: Developmental Trajectories and Implications

The emerging patterns are provocative, and suggest a coherent developmental trajectory. Early in development, mothers and fathers engage their young children in reminiscing about the emotional events of their lives, and this reminiscing is gendered. Mothers are more elaborative and more emotionally expressive than are fathers, and both mothers and fathers are more elaborative and emotionally expressive with daughters than with sons. Reminiscing is also placed in a more social relational context with daughters than with sons. Returning to the theoretical perspectives outlined at the beginning of this chapter, children are drawn into gendered reminiscing in ways that both model and mold their emerging autobiographical voice. Girls are learning to narrate their own emotional lives in more elaborated and emotionally expressive ways than are boys, and we see these differences as children become more competent narrators of their personal past through middle childhood and adolescence.

As adults, these gendered patterns continue, and extend to the family [Bohanek et al., 2009; Buckner & Fivush, 2000; Fivush et al., 2010]. Females (mothers) tell more elaborated and more emotionally expressive narratives than do males (fathers). Children are exposed to both gendered reminiscing about their own personal experiences and those of their parents. Thus, the cycle repeats, with parents modeling and molding the next generation into gendered reminiscing. Importantly, it is not that boys do not know how to tell elaborated and emotionally expressive narratives; they can do so when telling stories about their mother's childhoods. Rather, the argument is that through socially structured parentally guided interactions, children are learning to value reminiscing in particular ways over others. For boys, the emotional past is more about the facts of what happened. For girls, the emotional past is about feelings and about relationships. Thus, the emotional past defines us in gendered ways.

Moreover, gendered reminiscing has implications for evolving emotional well-being. Early in development, mothers who are more elaborative and emotionally expressive help their children to better understand and regulate their own emotional lives. We have too little research on fathers to draw any conclusions, and the little we have is difficult to interpret. This is a critical avenue for future research. As children develop into adolescence, we begin to see gender differences in relations between gendered reminiscing and well-being. Although girls are narrating personal stories that are more elaborate and emotionally expressive than are boys, there are no relations to their emotional well-being. In contrast, although boys are telling more factual narratives overall, those boys who include more emotional expression show higher emotional well-being. Yet, consistent with girls being more relationally oriented in understanding their emotional lives, those girls who tell stories about their mothers childhoods that are more emotionally expressive show higher levels of emotional well-being, whereas there are no relations for girls to paternal intergenerational narratives, nor any relations for boys. That adolescent males and females tell different kinds of stories about themselves and about their parents, and that there are differential relations to emotional well-being confirms that this is not a general effect of narrative ability or between narratives and well-being. Rather, adolescents are choosing to tell personal stories that reflect a gendered understanding of self. It is in this sense that adolescents are developing an emotional voice. That this voice is differentially related to emotional well-being is intriguing and deserves additional research attention.

References

Adams, S., Kuebli, J., Boyle, P.A., & Fivush, R. (1995). Gender differences in parent-child conversations about past emotions: A longitudinal investigation. *Sex Roles, 33*, 309.

Bauer, P., Stennes, L., & Haight, J. (2003). Representation of the inner self in autobiography: Women's and men's use of internal states language in personal narratives. *Memory, 11*, 27–42.

Belenky, M.F., Clinchy, B.M., Goldberger, N.R., & Tarule, J.M. (1986). *Women's ways of knowing: The development of self, voice and mind.* New York: Basic Books.

Bird, A., & Reese, E. (2006). Emotional reminiscing and the development of an autobiographical self. *Developmental Psychology, 42*, 613–626.

Bohanek, J.G., & Fivush, R. (2010). Personal narratives, well-being, and gender in adolescence. *Cognitive Development, 25*, 368–379.

Bohanek, J.G., Fivush, R., Zaman, W., Lepore, C., Merchant, S., & Duke, P. (2009). Narrative interaction in family dinnertime conversations: Relations to child well-being. *Merrill Palmer Quarterly, 55*, 488–515.

Bohanek, J.G., Marin, K., & Fivush, R. (2008). Family narratives, self, and gender in early adolescence. *The Journal of Early Adolescence, 28*, 153–176.

Bordo, S. (1990). Feminism, postmodernism and gender skepticism. In L. Nicholson (Ed.), *Feminism/Postmodernism* (pp. 133–156). New York: Routledge.

Brody, L.R., & Hall, J.A. (2008). Gender and emotion in context. In M. Lewis, J.M. Haviland-Jones & L. Feldman-Barrett (Eds.), *Handbook of emotions. Vol. 3* (pp. 395–408). New York: Guilford Press.

Bruner, J.S. (1990). *Acts of meaning*. Cambridge: Harvard University Press.

Buckner, J.P., & Fivush, R. (2000). Gendered themes in family reminiscing. *Memory, 8*, 401–412.

Buckner, J.P., & Fivush, R. (1998). Gender and self in children's autobiographical narratives. *Applied Cognitive Psychology, 12*, 407–429.

Cross, S.E., & Madson, L. (1997). Models of the self: Self-construals and gender. *Psychological Bulletin, 122*, 5–37.

Dunn, J., Brown, J., & Beardsall, L. (1991). Family talk about feeling states and children's later understanding of others' emotions. *Developmental Psychology, 27*, 448–455.

Eisenberg, N., Spinrad, T.L., & Eggum, N.D. (2010). Emotion-related self-regulation and its relations to children's maladjustment. *Annual Review of Psychology, 6*, 495–525.

Fiese, B.H., & Bickham, N.L. (2004). Pin-curling grandpa's hair in the comfy chair: Parents' stories of growing up and potential links to socialization in the preschool years. In M.W. Pratt & B.H. Fiese (Eds.), *Family stories and the life course* (pp. 259–277). Mahwah: Lawrence Erlbaum Associates, Inc.

Fiese, B.H., & Skillman, G. (2000). Gender differences in family stories: Moderating influence of parent gender role and child gender. *Sex Roles, 43*, 267–283.

Fischer, A.H., & Manstead, A.R. (2008). Social functions of emotions. In M. Lewis, J.M. Haviland-Jones & L. Feldman-Barrett (Eds.), *Handbook of emotions. Vol. 3* (pp. 456–468). New York: Guilford Press.

Fivush, R. (1989). Exploring sex differences in the emotional content of mother-child conversations about the past. *Sex Roles, 20*, 675–691.

Fivush, R. (2004). Voice and silence: A feminist model of autobiographical memory. In J.M. Lucariello, J.A. Hudson, R. Fivush & P.J. Bauer (Eds.), *The development of the mediated mind* (pp. 79–100). Mahwah: Lawrence Erlbaum.

Fivush, R. (2007). Maternal reminiscing style and children's developing understanding of self and emotion. *Clinical Social Work, 35*, 37–46.

Fivush, R. (2010). Speaking Silence: The social construction of voice and silence in cultural and autobiographical narratives. *Memory, 18*, 88–98.

Fivush, R., Berlin, L.J., Sales, J.M., Mennuti-Washburn, J., Cassidy, J. (2003). Functions of parent-child reminiscing about emotionally negative events. *Memory, 11*, 179–192.

Fivush, R., Bohanek, J.G., & Duke, M. (2005). The intergenerational self: Subjective perspective and family history. In F. Sani (Ed.), *Individual and collective self-continuity*. Mahwah: Lawrence Erlbaum Associates, Inc.

Fivush, R., Bohanek, J.G., Marin, K., & Duke, M. (2010). Family narratives and adolescent well-being. In K.C. McLean & M. Pasupathi (Eds.). *Narrative Development in Adolescence: Creating the Storied Self* (pp. 45–64). NY: Springer.

Fivush, R., Bohanek, J.G., Zaman, W., & Grapin, S. (2011). Gender differences in adolescent's autobiographical narratives. *Journal of Cognitive Development, 13*, 295–319.

Fivush, R., Brotman, M.A., Buckner, J.P., & Goodman, S.H. (2000). Gender differences in parent-child emotion narratives. *Sex Roles, 42*, 233–253.

Fivush, R., & Buckner, J.P. (2003). Constructing gender and identity through autobiographical narratives. In R. Fivush & C. Haden (Eds.), *Autobiographical memory and the construction of a narrative self: Developmental and cultural perspectives* (pp. 149–168). Mahwah: Erlbaum.

Fivush, R., Haden, C.A., & Reese, E. (2006). Elaborating on elaborations: Maternal reminiscing style and children's socio-emotional outcome. *Child Development, 77*, 1568–1588.

Fivush, R., Marin, K., McWilliams, K., & Bohanek, J.G. (2009). Family reminiscing style: Parent gender and emotional focus in relation to child well-being. *Journal of Cognition and Development, 10*, 210–235.

Fivush, R., & Nelson, K. (2004). Culture and language in the emergence of autobiographical memory. *Psychological Science, 15*, 586–590.

Fivush, R., & Zaman, W. (in press). Gender, subjectivity and autobiography. In P.J. Bauer & R. Fivush (Eds.), *Handbook of the Development of Children's Memory.* New York: Wiley-Blackwell.

Gergen, M. (2001). Feminist reconstructions in psychology: Narrative gender and performance. New York: Sage.

Gilligan, C. (1982). In a different voice: Psychological theory and women's development. Cambridge: Harvard University Press.

Haden, C.A., & Fivush, R. (1996). Contextual variation in maternal conversational styles. *Merrill-Palmer Quarterly, 42*, 200–227. http://www.jstor.org/stable/23087877.

Harris, P.L. (2008). Children's understanding of emotion. In M. Lewis, J.M. Haviland-Jones & L. Feldman-Barrett (Eds.), *Handbook of emotions. Vol. 3* (pp. 320–331). New York: Guilford Press.

Kuebli, J., & Fivush, R. (1992). Gender differences in parent-child conversations about past emotions. *Sex Roles, 27*, 683–698.

Kuebli, J., Butler, S., & Fivush, R. (1995). Mother-child talk about past emotions: Relations of maternal language and child gender overtime. In J. Dunn (Ed.), *Connections between emotion and understanding in development.* (pp. 265–284). London: Lawrence Erlbaum Associates.

Kulkofsky, S., Wang, Q., & Kim Koh, J.B. (2009). Functions of memory sharing and mother-child reminiscing behaviors: Individual and cultural variations. *Journal of Cognition and Development, 10*, 92–114.

Lagattuta, K.H., & Wellman, H.M. (2002). Differences in early parent-child conversations about negative vs. positive emotions: Implications for the development of psychological understanding. *Developmental Psychology, 38*, 564–589.

Laible, D. (2004). Mother-child discourse in two contexts: Links with child temperament, attachment security, and socio-emotional competence. *Developmental Psychology, 40*, 979–992.

Lazarus, R.S. (2006). Emotions and interpersonal relationships: Toward a person-centered conceptualization of emotions and coping. *Journal of Personality, 74*, 9–46.

McAdams, D.P. (2001). The psychology of life stories. *Review of General Psychology, 5*, 100–122.

McLean, K., Pasupathi, M., & Pals, J. (2007). Selves creating stories creating selves: A process model of self-development. *Personality and Social Psychology Review, 11*, 262–278.

Merrill, N., Walsh, K., Zaman, W., & Fivush, R. (2011) *Coherence across adolescents' personal and intergenerational narratives.* Paper presented at the biennial meetings of the Society for Research in Child Development, Montreal, Canada.

Niedzwienska, A. (2003). Gender differences in vivid memories. *Sex Roles, 49*, 321–331.

Nolen-Hoeksema, S., Wisco, B.E., & Lyubomirsky, S. (2008). Rethinking rumination. *Perspectives on Psychological Science, 3*, 400–424.

Norris, J.E., Kuiack, S., & Pratt, M.W. (2004). 'As long as the go back down the driveway at the end of the day': Stories of the satisfactions and challenges on grandparenthood. In M.W. Pratt & B.H. Fiese (Eds.), *Family stories and the life course: Across time and generations* (pp. 353–373). Mahwah: Erlbaum.

Pasupathi, M., & Wainryb, C. (2010). On telling the whole story: Facts and interpretations in autobiographical memory narratives from childhood through mid-adolescence. *Developmental Psychology, 46*, 735–746.

Reese, E., & Cleveland, E. (2006). Mother-child reminiscing and children's understanding of mind. *Merrill-Palmer Quarterly, 52*, 17–43.

Reese, E., & Fivush, R. (1993). Parental styles of talking about the past. *Developmental Psychology, 29*, 596–606.

Reese, E., Haden, C.A., & Fivush, R. (1996). Mothers, fathers, daughters, sons: Gender differences in autobiographical reminiscing. *Research on Language and Social Interaction, 29*, 27–56.

Reese, E., Haden, C.A., & Fivush, R. (1993). Mother-child conversations about the past: Relationships of style and memory over time. *Cognitive Development, 8*, 403–430.

Reese, E., & Newcombe, R. (2007). Training mothers in elaborative reminiscing enhances children's autobiographical memory and narrative. *Child Development, 78*, 1153–1170.

Reese, E., Yan, C., Jack, F., & Hayne, H. (2010). Emerging identities: Narrative and self from early childhood to early adolescence. In K. McLean & M. Pasupathi (Eds.), *Narrative development in adolescence: Creating the storied self* (pp. 23–43). New York: Springer.

Rime, B. (2007). The social sharing of emotion as an interface between individual and collective processes in the construction of emotional climate. *Journal of Social Issues, 63*, 307–322.

Rose, A.J., Carlson, W., & Waller, E.M. (2007). Prospective associations of co-rumination with friendship and emotional adjustment: Considering the socioemotional tradeoffs of co-ruminations. *Developmental Psychology, 43*, 1019–1031.

Rosser, S.V., & Miller, P.J. (2000). Feminist theories: Implications for developmental psychology. In P. Miller & E. Scholnick (Eds.), *Towards a feminist developmental psychology* (pp. 11–28). New York: Cambridge University Press.

Saarni, C. (2008). The interface of emotional development and social context. In M. Lewis, J.M. Haviland-Jones & L. Feldman-Barrett (Eds.), *Handbook of emotions. Vol. 3* (pp. 332–347). New York: Guilford Press.

Sales, J.M., Fivush, R., & Peterson, C. (2003). Parental reminiscing about positive and negative events. *Journal of Cognition and Development, 42*, 185–209.

Vygotsky, L.S. (1978). Mind in society: The development of higher psychological processes. Cambridge: Harvard University Press.

Wang, Q. (in press). The cultured self and remembering. In P.J. Bauer & R. Fivush (Eds.), *Handbook of the Development of Children's Memory*. New York: Wiley-Blackwell.

Wang, Q., Doan, S.N., & Song, Q. (2010). Talking about internal states in mother-child reminiscing influences children's self-representations: A cross-cultural study. *Cognitive Development, 25*, 380–393.

Welch-Ross, M.K., Fasig, L., & Farrar, M.J. (1999). Predictors of preschoolers' self-knowledge: Reference to emotion and mental states in mother-child conversation about past events. *Cognitive Development, 14*, 401–422.

Widen, S.C., & Russell, J.A. (2008). Young children's understanding of others' emotions. In M. Lewis, J.M. Haviland-Jones & L. Feldman-Barrett (Eds.), *Handbook of emotions. Vol. 3* (pp. 348–363). New York: Guilford Press.

Zaman, W., & Fivush, R. (2011). When my mom was a little girl...: Gender differences in adolescents' intergenerational and personal narratives. *Journal of Research on Adolescence*. DOI: 10.1111/j.1532–7795.2010.00709.x.

Zaman, W., & Fivush, R. (in press). Gender differences in parent-child reminiscing about emotional and play events. *Sex Roles*.

Robyn Fivush
Department of Psychology
Emory University
Atlanta, GA 30322 (USA)
E-Mail psyrf@emory.edu

Hansen Lagattuta K (ed): Children and Emotion. New Insights into Developmental Affective Sciences.
Contrib Hum Dev. Basel, Karger, 2014, vol 26, pp 95–105 (DOI: 10.1159/000354362)

How Does Talk about Thoughts, Desires, and Feelings Foster Children's Socio-Cognitive Development? Mediators, Moderators and Implications for Intervention

Claire Hughes · Naomi White · Rosie Ensor

Centre for Family Research, Department of Psychology, University of Cambridge, Cambridge, UK

Abstract

Over the past two decades, research into social influences on young children's growing understanding of others' thoughts and feelings has highlighted the value of conversations. This chapter takes up this proposal and is divided into four sections. The first outlines converging evidence from studies of twins, studies of children with hearing impairments, and longitudinal studies of typically developing children that children's linguistic environments contribute to their socio-cognitive development. The second section identifies two alternative mediators of this relationship: semantic versus pragmatic aspects of maternal scaffolding. The third section considers moderating influences of social partner and culture. The fourth section illustrates how experimental training studies help to elucidate underlying mechanisms by revealing that children's understanding of mind and emotion can be enhanced through language-based interventions.

When investigations into children's understanding of mind first began more than three decades ago, a key research aim was to document and explain universal developmental mile-stones in children's understanding of their own and others' thoughts, desires and feelings [e.g., Bartsch & Wellman, 1995]. As a result, the studies involved a limited set of tasks and small homogeneous samples (typically, middle class 3- to 5-year-olds). A second wave of research developed a wider array of tasks and included larger, more diverse samples, revealing striking individual differences in children's understanding of mind. Key social influences were identified, including both distal factors (e.g., family size, maternal education) and proximal factors (e.g., attachment security, linguistic environment). Over the past decade, a third wave of studies has seen a dramatic expansion in the developmental scope of this research, including a raft of new studies of infants and a small but growing body of work on mindreading in older children, adolescents, and adults. This third wave of research has also enhanced our understanding of social influences on children's social understanding and the importance of both context and culture.

We begin by outlining the case for a causal relation between children's socio-linguistic environments and their social understanding (i.e., their understanding of mental states such as beliefs and emotions). Next we consider the insights that have emerged from studies of mediators and moderators of this relation with respect to one particular social influence: family talk about desires, thoughts, and feelings. Finally, we discuss training studies as well as clinical implications of research in this field.

Is Variation in Children's Socio-Linguistic Environments Causally Related to Variation in Social Understanding?

Comparing identical and fraternal twins for similarity in any given trait serves as a simple natural experiment for assessing the relative magnitude of genetic and environmental effects. Interestingly, existing twin findings suggest that as children get older environmental influences on individual differences in understanding of mind become increasingly salient. Specifically, a study of 119 pairs of 3-year-old same-sex twins highlights the importance of genetic influences [Hughes & Cutting, 1999], but findings from two studies of older children provide compelling evidence for environmental influences on individual differences in school-aged children's understanding of mind. The first of these involved a large and representative community sample of 1,116 same-sex 5-year-old twin pairs who completed a battery of tasks (including classic false-belief tasks, prediction of emotion from false-belief tasks and second order false-belief tasks) and showed that non-genetic factors accounted for 93% of the variance in total scores [Hughes et al., 2005]. The second study involved 388 pairs of 9-year-old same-sex twins who completed an advanced test of theory of mind (the Strange Stories [Happé, 1994]) and showed that 88% of variation in task scores could be attributed to non-genetic factors [Ronald, Viding, Happé & Plomin, 2006]. Note that these studies involved different tasks and different age groups and yet both showed a robust effect of environment on individual differences in understanding of mind.

Another natural experiment that highlights the importance of conversation for children's understanding of mind is the comparison of early- versus late-signing children with hearing impairments. This (much larger) latter group of children do not have normal access to conversational interactions and are severely delayed in their performance on theory-of-mind tasks [e.g., Peterson & Siegal, 1998]. Importantly, this contrast remains significant even in studies that involve early-/late-signing groups of hearing impaired children who are matched for linguistic competence [Woolfe, Want & Siegal, 2002]. Although it does not preclude an important role for children's own language acquisition in the development of an understanding of mind [c.f., Astington & Baird, 2005], this finding does provide good evidence for the importance of early exposure to rich conversational interactions.

Alongside the vast number of experimental studies of children's understanding of mind, the past three decades have also seen a much smaller but sustained parallel strand of research into young children's talk about thoughts and feelings. This observational research began with a landmark study by Bretherton and Beeghly [1982]. Subsequent work by Bartsch and Wellman [1995], who sampled from ten children in the CHILDES study between the ages of 2 and 5 years to examine more than 200,000 everyday conversations, revealed sequences in children's talk about desires, emotions, beliefs and thoughts that are comparable to the milestones identified in experimental research. Later research by Lagattuta and Wellman [2002] further revealed significant gains between 2 and 5 years of age in the frequency of talk about causes and consequences of emotions as well as connections between emotions and other mental states in both children's and parents' everyday conversations.

Interest in children's exposure to talk about mental states was sparked by Dunn and colleagues' documentation of specific predictive associations between family discourse about mental states and emotions and children's later success on tests of false belief and emotion understanding [e.g., Dunn, Brown & Beardsall, 1991]. However, the aggregate approach adopted in these studies made it impossible to assess whether exposure to mental-state talk from family members showed independent effects on children's later social understanding. To tackle this issue, Ruffman, Slade and Crowe [2002] adopted a cross-lagged longitudinal design in a lab-based study of 82 2- to 4-year-olds that included direct measures of children's verbal skills and both mothers' and children's mental-state references, including talk about emotions, while looking at photos at each of 3 time-points across 12 months. Their findings showed impressive stability in mothers' mental state discourse over the three time periods. Over and above associations with non-mental discourse, mothers who referred to mental states more at earlier time points had children who later scored higher on the theory-of-mind tasks. This predictive relationship remained even when earlier child theory of mind, child linguistic ability, and child mental state utterances were all taken into account. These findings provide compelling evidence for a causal relation between maternal mental-state talk and children's social understanding.

Space does not allow us to summarize all the individual studies [at least 30 are noted in a recent review by Pavarini, de Hollanda Souza & Hawk, 2013]; instead, we shall focus on a handful of studies that stand apart from the field in particular ways. The first of these is Jenkins et al.'s [2003] longitudinal study. They included an exceptionally large corpus based on 9 h of interactions for each of 37 children, encompassing both dyadic interactions with mothers and multi-partner interactions involving fathers and older siblings (discussed in more detail later in this chapter). Their findings revealed interesting contrasts between conversations about distinct mental states. For example, family talk about cognitive and feeling states at child age 2 predicted changes in children's cognitive and feeling talk, respectively, across a 2-year interval. These specific predictive relations remained significant when initial levels of child talk and children's general language ability were taken into account. Increases in children's cognitive talk between the ages of 2 and 4 were more striking than increases in talk about desires or feelings; moreover, older siblings' cognitive talk also increased from ages 4 to 6, whereas desire and feeling talk decreased. Together, these findings highlight the potential importance of talk about cognitive states in particular. Indeed, other studies have shown that maternal references to cognitions are a particularly consistent correlate of children's false-belief understanding [Ensor & Hughes, 2008; Slaughter, Peterson & MacKintosh, 2007]. One reason for this may be that cognitive states, unlike desires or emotions, rarely have corresponding behavioural or facial cues [Bartsch & Wellman, 1995].

In another distinctive study, involving 120 mother-child dyads followed from age 2 to age 4, Ensor and Hughes [2008] examined both conversational content (e.g., talk about distinct mental states – cognition, desire, emotion) and quality (e.g., connected, initiatory, failed, and conflictual turns) at age 2. The authors aimed to assess whether these measures showed independent or interacting associations with gains in children's performance on tests of social understanding over this 2-year period. Their findings demonstrated that all three types of mental-state talk occurred especially frequently within connected turns; confirming the particular importance of connected talk about cognitive states.

Two further studies are distinctive by virtue of their extended developmental and temporal scope. Whereas most studies have focused heavily on preschoolers and involved relatively short temporal intervals, these three studies have examined relations between maternal mental-state talk and children's mental-state awareness across relatively long intervals that bridge preschool research and studies of both infants and school-aged children. The first two of these studies demonstrated that maternal sensitivity to infants' internal states predicted children's performance on mentalizing tasks approximately 4 years later. Specifically, Meins et al. [2003] found that mothers' appropriate mental-state comments during free play with their infants at 6 months, including talk about the infants' emotions, predicted children's performance on a stream-of-consciousness task at age 55 months (n = 52). An interpretation here is that mothers' appropriate comments on their infants' mental states provide a linguistic and conceptual scaffold in which infants' attention is drawn to the existence and functional significance of mental states and processes [Meins et al., 2003].

In the second study to provide a compelling case for the importance of mothers' early talk about mental states, Ensor, Devine and Hughes [2012] showed that individual differences in the frequencies of mothers' references to cognitive states, recorded at child ages 2 and 6: (a) were stable across a 4-year period, (b) predicted children's false-belief understanding 4 years later even when both this stability of individual differences in mothers' cognitive references and children's initial false-belief understanding were taken into account, and (c) predicted children's success on the Strange Stories at age 10 – that is, as much as 8 years later.

What Mediates the Relation between Talk about Thoughts and Feelings and Children's Understanding of Belief and Emotion?

Theoretical accounts of what might mediate the association between family talk and children's understanding of belief and emotion come in at least two flavours. The first of these fits within a Vygotskian perspective in which language is a key vehicle for the transmission of knowledge [Vygotsky, 1962] and highlights the semantic information included within conversational references to thoughts and feelings. As argued by Taumoepeau and Ruffman [2008], one plausible account is that maternal language acts as a zone of proximal development for children's cognitive development – beginning with desire words, mothers gradually introduce their children to more abstract cognitive terms (e.g., think, know). Ruffman, Taumoepeau and Perkins [2012] note features of maternal input that serve to assist children's prediction of people's actions and understanding of the social world. For example, by referring to a particular mental state within multiple contexts, mothers help children (at least eventually) to understand that this term cannot refer to a specific behaviour or context.

Interestingly, while a recent re-examination of longitudinal data has enabled Meins et al. [in press] to provide empirical support for the perspective summarised above, the same analysis also revealed support for an alternative account, in which maternal talk about thoughts and feelings is held to facilitate the growth of children's social understanding through its pragmatic function of highlighting differences in points of view [Harris, de-Rosnay & Pons, 2005]. Specifically, Meins et al. [in press] found that mothers who made frequent 'non-attuned' comments about their 8-month-olds' mental states had children who performed poorly on theory-of-mind tasks at 51 months and this association was mediated by low levels of perspectival symbolic play at 26 months.

At this point it is worth noting that it is entirely possible to highlight differences in points of view without explicit reference to thoughts or beliefs. Similarly, parents and children often emotionally evaluate conversational content without explicitly commenting on how they feel (e.g., by laughing). Take, for example, this excerpt from a conversation between a mother and her 8-year-old son (reproduced from Hughes [2011]):

Mother: Has anyone been getting up to mischief today Lucas? Any good stories? Anybody put the shower on your clothes today? (smiles)

Lucas: No, not today. (laughs)

Mother: So has anyone got to the bottom of what happened then?

Lucas: Probably, but I haven't heard.

Mother: Okay, so they haven't expelled any third formers yet then?

Lucas: Nobody's been expelled, but they're in deep trouble.

Here the mother steers the conversation into waters that are rich in reference to points of view (shared reference to an earlier conversation, changes in knowledge states, and heavy handed disciplinary action in response to student mischief) – all without actually using any mental state terms. That said, the next few turns in the above conversation did in fact include several diverse and explicit references to cognitive states (underlined):

Lucas: Strangely, the teacher <u>didn't even know</u> where the switch was, Mr. Mason

Mother: So he couldn't turn it off? (disbelief and amusement)

Lucas: Yes. Me and Richard had to go in there with our clothes on. (laughs)

Mother: (Laughs) Getting soaked. Oh no. Who was in the changing room? I bet everyone was really laughing. What did Douglas say?

Lucas: Soaked.

Mother: He got soaked. I <u>bet he thought</u> that was hilarious, didn't he? (smiling)

In other words, echoing Ensor and Hughes [2008] finding that naturally occurring talk about cognitive states appeared particularly frequently within connected conversations, mental-state references may simply be a good proxy for high quality (i.e., connected, elaborative) conversations that are likely to foster children's pragmatic awareness of differences in points of view. This leads us neatly into the next section, which considers potential moderators of the relationship between family talk and improvements in children's social understanding.

What Moderates the Relationship between Talk and Social Understanding?

Existing research on the contribution of family talk to children's social understanding has focused almost exclusively on conversations with mothers and has typically involved white middle class families, constraining the conclusions that can be drawn. In this section, we examine whether links between family talk and children's social understanding differ for conversations with other family members (siblings and fathers) or for families from different cultural backgrounds.

The nearly exclusive focus on talk with mothers is rather surprising because, by the age of 4 years, children engage in talk about thoughts and feelings more often with siblings than with mothers [Brown & Dunn, 1992]. One reason for this may be that children refer to cognitions, desires, and emotions preferentially within pretend play [Hughes, Fujisawa, Ensor, Lecce & Marfleet, 2006]. Note also that while mother-child mental state talk tends to focus on the child's desires, thoughts and feelings, sibling conversations are more likely to refer to both children's mental states [Brown & Dunn, 1992]. Talk about others' (rather than one's own) thoughts and feelings may be particularly important in children's early social understanding [Hughes, Lecce & Wilson, 2007].

Despite evidence for concurrent associations between children's mental state talk with siblings and theory of mind performance [e.g., Brown, Donelan-McCall & Dunn, 1996; Hughes et al., 2007] the longitudinal data needed to establish a causal influence are lacking. However, in a study of young friends, Hughes and Dunn [1998] showed that preschoolers' talk about thoughts and feelings predicted theory of mind performance 13 months later. This finding challenges the traditional Vygotskian emphasis on vertical interactions with cognitively more advanced social partners (e.g., caregivers). On this point it is worth noting that siblings may also contribute indirectly to children's theory of mind development by providing opportunities for the child to 'eavesdrop' on advanced conversations between a parent and an older child [Ruffman, Perner, Naito, Parkin & Clements, 1998]. Supporting this idea, Jenkins et al. [2003] found that 4-year-olds with an older sibling were exposed to more cognitive talk than 4-year-olds with a younger sibling, and much of this talk occurred between parents and children rather than between the children themselves. Similarly, in a recent training study Gola [2012, discussed in more detail later in this chapter] found improvements in children's false-belief understanding when children overheard cognitive state talk (think, know, remember) about others. These findings emphasize the importance of exposure to, as well as participation in, conversations about mental states, and they echo the themes that emerge from research on mother-child mental state talk.

Fathers' talk has also been neglected in investigations of children's developing social understanding. The few studies that include fathers suggest interesting differences between fathers' and mothers' mental state talk. Fathers appear to make fewer references to emotions and cognitions than mothers, in picture-book reading tasks [LaBounty, Wellman, Olson, Lagattuta & Liu, 2008], and in conversations about emotionally-valenced past events [Bohanek, Marin & Fivush, 2008; Fivush, Brotman, Buckner & Goodman, 2000; see also Fivush, this vol.]. However, this contrast may be restricted to tasks that explicitly prime emotion talk: Mothers and fathers do not seem to differ in their references to emotion during conversations about more general past events [e.g., Kuebli & Fivush, 1992], perhaps because of the infrequency of emotion references in naturally occurring conversations [McElwain, Booth-LaForce & Wu, 2011].

Moreover, the study by LaBounty et al. [2008] highlighted differences in the relationship between mothers' and fathers' talk and children's social understanding. Specifically, mothers' (but not fathers') emotion talk predicted 3.5-year-olds' concurrent emotion understanding. Fathers' explanatory talk about desires, however, predicted children's performance on false belief tasks, both concurrently and 18 months later. These findings suggest differential roles for parents in children's lives. For example, Bhavnagri and Parke [1991] have suggested that fathers take on more of a 'playmate' role than mothers. More work is needed to address this hypothesis.

Culture may also play a large part in children's social understanding: the values of a society shape parental practices and expectations for children's behaviour [see Camras et al., this vol.]. Of particular relevance to this chapter is the growing body of research that suggests that Chinese-American mothers appear to use more emotion attributions, but fewer explanations than their European-American counterparts when talking with children about past events [Fivush & Wang, 2005; Wang & Fivush, 2005]. Differences in mothers' mental state talk probably reflect core values of collectivist versus individualistic societies. In Western cultures, social relationships are largely voluntary and talk about emotions in past events is an important way of bonding with others and maintaining close relationships [Wang, 2008]. Conversely, in Chinese culture, relationships are influenced by established roles and hierarchies [Hsu, 1953] and thus emotion talk may be less crucial in maintaining relationships. Challenging this view, however, another study has shown that a predictive link between mothers' mental-state talk in a picture-book task and children's emotion understanding for both Chinese-American mothers and European-American mothers [Doan & Wang, 2010].

Working with different cultural groups, Garrett-Peters et al. [2008, 2011] have found differences between African-American and non-African-American families in both the frequency and the correlates of parents' emotion talk. Similarly, Eisenberg [1999] has shown that Mexican-American mothers refer to others' emotions more frequently than European-American mothers [c.f., Hughes et al., 2007]. However, more detailed investigations of other cultures, as well as studies of native and immigrant families, are still needed. For example, Chinese mothers living in the US exhibit a more 'Chinese' pattern of mental state talk during past event talk and storytelling than mothers living in China [Wang, 2012]. Similarly, differences in emotion talk between first- and second-generation Mexican families living in the US have also been documented [Cervantes, 2002]. As societies become increasingly multi-cultural, it is vital that researchers not only include non-European families in their studies of family influences, but also that they adopt a more nuanced approach that includes, for example, contrasts both between particular ethnic groups and between first- and second-generation immigrant families.

Implications for Interventions: Training Studies and the Predictive Utility of Variation in Social Understanding

Beyond their value as a real-life application of research, training studies provide an important means of testing theories. In particular, data from training studies are critical for assessing the causal impact of conversational input because child-driven effects mean that correlations between maternal talk and children's later socio-cognitive performance may simply reflect stable within-child characteristics. In one of the first training studies, Slaughter and Gopnik [1996] found improved performance for children who received training on the concepts of either belief or desire and perception (but not for a control group who received training on number conservation). These results highlight the socio-cognitive benefits of discourse about mental states, and they suggest that children hold a coherent intuitive theory of mind from as early as 3 years of age.

In a later study, Lohmann and Tomasello [2003] included four different groups to tease apart effects of training in a specific aspect of language, sentential complements (e.g., 'This boy said that X') from more general discourse about deceptive situations. Their findings provide compelling evidence for the importance of language. Specifically, compared with children trained in non-verbal deceptive situations, post-test false-belief scores were higher for children trained in: (a) (non-deceptive) sentential complements; (b) perspective-discourse about deceptive situations, or (c) both sentential complements and perspective discourse. Moreover, despite receiving the same contact time with the experimenters, the third group outperformed the other two linguistic training groups, suggesting that training in sentential complementation and perspective-taking discourse each independently assist children's false-belief understanding.

Recently, Gola [2012] has also reported gains in false-belief understanding for children who, rather than receiving direct training with feedback, were simply asked to watch video clips involving mental verb utterances that varied in form (statement or question), referent (first person or other person), or style (overheard or direct). This simple exposure approach greatly increases the accessibility of training and provides a useful bridge between the results from training studies and studies involving naturalistic observations of family conversations. These findings further highlight the benefits of 'eavesdropping' on discourse about mental states [Jenkins et al., 2003]. What is not yet known, however, is whether the impact of linguistic environments is constrained by child characteristics, such as the ability to shift attention (in order to either listen in on a conversation, or to appreciate differences in points of view [c.f., Russell, 1997; Sabbagh, Hopkins, Benson & Flanagan, 2010]).

Extending the above work with preschool samples, others have begun to assess whether training can also facilitate social understanding beyond the preschool years. For example, Lecce et al. [2012] conducted an intervention study in which a trained researcher led carefully matched groups of 9-year-olds in discussions of either mentalistic or physical vignettes (based on Happé's [1994] Strange Stories task). The significant group difference at post-test was maintained over a 2-month follow-up and transferred to a novel task involving silent film clips [Devine & Hughes, 2013]. In a separate study, Goldstein and Winner [2012] have examined whether training in acting (which involves 'stepping into others' shoes') is more effective than training in visual arts or music at improving empathic accuracy. Positive results were found for adolescents but not younger children; training intensity was quite different for these groups (5–9 h vs. 90 min a week), suggesting a possible dosage effect. Taken together, these two studies demonstrate plasticity in typically-developing individuals' theory-of-mind skills that extends well beyond the preschool years.

Returning to the question of what training studies might achieve, one obvious question concerns whether children with autism, who show marked impairments in social understanding [Baron-Cohen, 2000] can be helped by theory-of-mind training. There are, of course, obvious constraints to note; in particular, conversation-based interventions are only appropriate for high-functioning individuals with autism. Moreover, while it is generally agreed that interventions should be delivered as early as possible, most very young children with autism have yet to develop functional language. In addition, while several studies (including a recent randomized controlled trial [Begeer et al., 2011]) have shown that children with autism can be trained to pass false-belief tasks [e.g., Fisher & Happé, 2005], the same studies typically also show that benefits do not generalize to improvements in children's social or conversational skills.

Here it is worth noting that the dosage effect invoked by Goldstein and Winner [2012] may apply a fortiori to individuals with autism, for whom extensive (and repetitive) conversational experience may be necessary to acquire and strengthen an understanding of mind. In particular, it may be that impairments in executive function, which also appear characteristic of children with autism [Hill, 2004], limit their ability to shift attention between conversational partners or topics; decreasing the likelihood of benefitting from enriched conversational environments. Thus, one promising direction for future research would be to investigate moderating effects of executive function on the relation between conversational input and social understanding in both typically developing children and children with autism. Another means of facilitating improvements in understanding of mind among children with autism might be to focus on internal states that can be made salient more readily than cognitions – such as emotions. Support for this approach comes from the finding that while typically developing children's performance on false-belief tasks is associated with mothers' use of explanatory, causal and contrastive talk about cognition, children with autism's performance on false belief tasks is uniquely correlated with mothers' use of explanatory, causal and contrastive talk about emotion [Slaughter et al., 2007].

Conversational training also appears feasible and worthwhile in other clinical groups, such as children with conduct problems, who are more likely than their peers to display a hostile attribution bias [for a meta-analysis, see de Castro, Veerman, Koops, Bosch & Monshouwer, 2002]. This hostile attribution bias may well be learned at home, as hostile appraisals in children and mothers appear significantly correlated [Root & Jenkins, 2005]. Thus, training mothers' in more positive forms of discourse may help to ameliorate childhood conduct problems. Supporting the feasibility of this approach, Salmon, Dadds, Allen and Hawes [2009] trained parents either to use elaborative, emotion-rich reminiscing or to allow their child to take the lead during play sessions. At post-test, results showed reduced oppositional behaviour in children in both conditions, but greater use of elaborations and emotion references in the interactions of parent-dyads given the emotion-talk training. Therefore, rather than focusing solely on reducing negative behaviors, interventions that promote positive family interactions may also help children with conduct problems.

Training studies have, to date, been largely focused on refining theoretical models of how children's social environments contribute to their growing understanding of mind, rather than on enhancing children's social or cognitive functioning by improving their understanding of mind. Addressing this latter goal will clearly require careful attention to factors that constrain this influence. To borrow a point made by Lohmann and Tomasello [2003, p. 48] in their commentary on Nelson et al.'s [2003] paper, 'Entering a Community of Minds,' rather than this entry being simply a 'gift' from the community, it is likely that the child must do work to unpack the gift. The fact that training on false-sign or card-sorting tasks produces gains in children's understanding of mind that are equivalent to direct training on false-belief situations further suggests that children's executive skills should not be overlooked when designing interventions to foster children's social understanding and improve their social or cognitive competence.

Conclusion

In sum, in this chapter we have discussed several strands of evidence for conversational influences on children's growing understanding of mental states such as belief and emotion. These include natural experiments (such as studies of twins, or of deaf children living with deaf vs. hearing parents), cross-lagged analyses (documenting predictive effects over long periods of time, up to 8 years in one study) and training studies (which demonstrate significant gains in performance on theory-of-mind tasks following both engagement in and simple exposure to talk about thoughts and feelings). We have also outlined possible mediators of this association, including discourse that is connected to the child's point of view and/or that draws the child's attention to differences in points of view. Finally, while most studies in this field focus on mother-child conversations in white middle class families, we have summarized findings from the small but growing number of studies that investigate the influence of children's conversations with other social partners (e.g., siblings, fathers) or include more diverse samples (e.g., studies of atypical groups or of ethnic minority families or families in non-Western cultures). Together, these findings suggest a much richer picture of social influence, with distinct processes being key for different conversational partners or groups. At the moment, this picture is only sketched out in broad brush-stroke; the challenge for future research is to illuminate in fine detail exactly how children learn about the world of thoughts and feelings from their conversations with others.

References

Astington, J.W., & Baird, J. (2005). Representational development and false-belief understanding. In J.W. Astington & J. Baird (Eds.), *Why language matters for theory of mind* (pp. 163–185). New York: Oxford University Press.

Baron-Cohen, S. (2000). Theory of mind and autism: A fifteen year review. In S. Baron-Cohen, H. Tager-Flusberg & D. Cohen (Eds.), *Understanding other minds: Perspectives from developmental cognitive neuroscience* (2nd ed.). Oxford: Oxford University Press.

Bartsch, K., & Wellman, H. (1995). *Children talk about the mind*. Oxford: Oxford University Press.

Begeer, S., Gevers, C., Clifford, P., Verhoeve, M., Kat, K., Hoddenbach, E., & Boer, F. (2011). Theory of mind training in children with autism: A randomized controlled trial. *Journal of Autism and Developmental Disorders, 41*, 997–1006.

Bhavnagri, N., & Parke, R. (1991). Parents as direct facilitators of children's peer relationships: Effects of age of child and sex of parent. *Journal of Social and Personal Relationships, 8*, 423–440.

Bohanek, J., Marin, K., & Fivush, R. (2008). Family narratives, self and gender in early adolescence. *Journal of Early Adolescence, 28*, 153–176.

Bretherton, I., & Beeghly, M. (1982). Talking about internal states: The acquistion of a theory of mind. *Developmental Psychology, 18*, 906–921.

Brown, J., Donelan-McCall, N., & Dunn, J. (1996). Why talk about mental states? The significance of children's conversations with friends, siblings, and mothers. *Child Development, 67*, 836–849.

Brown, J., & Dunn, J. (1992). Talk with your mother or your sibling? Developmental changes in early family conversations about feelings. *Child Development, 63*, 336–349.

Cervantes, C. (2002). Explanatory emotion talk in Mexican immigrant and Mexican American families. *Hispanic Journal of Behavioral Sciences, 24*, 138–163.

de Castro, B., Veerman, J., Koops, W., Bosch, J., & Monshouwer, H. (2002). Hostile attribution of intent and aggressive behavior: A meta-analysis. *Child Development, 73*, 916–934.

Devine, R., & Hughes, C. (2013). Silent films and strange stories: Theory of mind, gender and social experiences in middle childhood. *Child Development, 84*, 989–1003.

Doan, S., & Wang, Q. (2010). Maternal discussions of mental states and behaviors: Relations to emotion situation knowledge in European American and immigrant Chinese children. *Child Development, 81*, 1490–1503.

Dunn, J., Brown, J., & Beardsall, L. (1991). Family talk about feeling states and children's later understanding of others' emotions. *Developmental Psychology, 27*, 448–455.

Eisenberg, A. (1999). Emotion talk among Mexican American and Anglo American mothers and children from two social classes. *Merrill-Palmer Quarterly, 45*, 267–284.

Ensor, R., Devine, R., & Hughes, C. (in press). Early exposure to mothers' cognitive references predicts theory of mind at ages 6 and 10. To appear in Child Develpment.

Ensor, R., & Hughes, C. (2008). Content or Connectedness? Early family talk and theory of mind in the toddler and preschool Years. *Child Development, 79*, 201–216.

Fisher, N., & Happé, F. (2005). A training study of theory of mind and executive function in children with Autistic Spectrum Disorders. *Journal of Autism and Developmental Disorders, 35*, 757–771.

Fivush, R., Brotman, M., Buckner, J., & Goodman, S. (2000). Gender differences in parent-child emotion narratives. *Sex Roles, 42*, 233–253.

Fivush, R., & Wang, Q. (2005). Emotion talk in mother-child conversations of the shared past: The effects of culture, gender, and event valence. *Journal of Cognition and Development, 6*, 489–506.

Garrett-Peters, P., Mills-Koonce, R., Adkins, D., Vernon-Feagans, L., Cox, M., & Investigators, F. L. P. K. (2008). Early environmental correlates of maternal emotion talk. *Parenting: Science and Practice, 8*, 117–152.

Garrett-Peters, P., Mills-Koonce, R., Zerwas, S., Cox, M., & Vernon-Feagans, L. (2011). Fathers' early emotion talk: Associations with income, ethnicity, and family factors. *Journal of Marriage and Family, 73*, 335–353.

Gola, A. (2012). Mental verb input for promoting children's theory of mind: A training study. *Cognitive Development, 27*, 64–76.

Goldstein, T., & Winner, E. (2012). Enhancing empathy and theory of mind. *Journal of Cognition and Development, 13*, 19–37.

Happé, F. (1994). An advanced test of theory of mind: Understanding of story characters' thoughts and feelings by able autistic, mentally handicapped, and normal children and adults. *Journal of Autism and Development Disorders, 24*, 129–154.

Harris, P., de-Rosnay, M., & Pons, F. (2005). Language and children's understanding of mental states. *Current Directions in Psychological Science, 14*, 69–73.

Hill, E. (2004). Executive function in autism. *Trends in Cognitive Sciences, 8*, 26–32.

Hsu, F. (1953). *Americans and Chinese: Purpose and fulfillment in great civilizations.* New York: The Natural History Press.

Hughes, C. (2011). *Social Understanding, Social Lives: From toddlerhood through to the transition to school.* London: Psychology Press.

Hughes, C., & Cutting, A. (1999). Nature, nurture and individual differences in early understanding of mind. *Psychological Science, 10*, 429–432.

Hughes, C., & Dunn, J. (1998). Understanding mind and emotion: Longitudinal associations with mental-state talk between young friends. *Developmental Psychology, 34*, 1026–1037.

Hughes, C., Fujisawa, K., Ensor, R., Lecce, S., & Marfleet, R. (2006). Cooperation and Conversations about the Mind: A study of individual differences in two-year-olds and their siblings. *British Journal of Developmental Psychology, 24*, 53–72.

Hughes, C., Jaffee, S., Happé, F., Taylor, A., Caspi, A., & Moffitt, T. (2005). Origins of individual differences in theory of mind: From nature to nurture? *Child Development, 76*, 356–370.

Hughes, C., Lecce, S., & Wilson, C. (2007). 'Do you know what I want?' Preschoolers' talk about desires, thoughts and feelings in their conversations with sibs and friends. *Cognition and Emotion, 21*, 330–350.

Jenkins, J., Turrell, S., Kogushi, Y., Lollis, S., & Ross, H. (2003). A longitudinal investigation of the dynamics of mental state talk in families. *Child Development, 74*, 905–920.

Kuebli, J., & Fivush, R. (1992). Gender differences in parent-child conversations about past emotions. *Sex Roles, 27*, 683–698.

LaBounty, J., Wellman, H., Olson, S., Lagattuta, K., & Liu, D. (2008). Mothers' *and* fathers' use of internal state talk with their young children. *Social Development, 4*, 757–775.

Lagattuta, K.H., & Wellman, H.M. (2002). Differences in early parent-child conversations about negative versus positive emotions: Implications for the development of psychological understanding. *Developmental Psychology, 38*, 564–580.

Lecce, S., Bianco, F., Devine, R., Hughes, C., & Banerjee, R. (2012). *Promoting theory of mind in middle childhood: A training study.* Submitted.

Lohmann, H., & Tomasello, M. (2003). The role of language in the development of false belief understanding: A training study. *Child Development, 74*, 1130–1144.

McElwain, N., Booth-LaForce, C., & Wu, X. (2011). Infant-mother attachment and children's friendship quality: Maternal mental-state talk as an intervening mechanism. *Developmental Psychology, 47*, 1295–1311.

Meins, E., Fernyhough, C., Arnott, B., Leekam, S., & de Rosnay, M. (2013). Mind-mindedness and theory of mind: Mediating roles of language and perspectival symbolic play. *Child Development, 84*, 1777–1790.

Meins, E., Fernyhough, C., Wainwright, R., Clark Carter, D., Gupta, M., Fradley, E., & Tuckey, M. (2003). Pathways to understanding mind: Construct validity and predictive validity of maternal mind-mindedness. *Child Development, 74*, 1194–1211.

Nelson, K., Skwerer, D., Goldman, S., Henseler, S., Presler, N., & Walkenfeld, F. (2003). Entering a community of minds: An experiential approach to 'theory of mind'. *Human Development, 46,* 24–46.
Pavarini, G., de Hollanda Souza, D., & Hawk, C. (2013). Parental practices and theory of mind development. *Journal of Child and Family Studies, 22,* 844–853.
Peterson, C., & Siegal, M. (1998). Changing focus on the representational mind: Deaf, autistic and normal children's concepts of false photos, false drawings and false beliefs. *British Journal of Developmental Psychology, 16,* 301–320.
Ronald, A., Viding, E., Happé, F., & Plomin, R. (2006). Individual differences in theory of mind ability in middle childhood and links with verbal ability and autistic traits: A twin study. *Social Neuroscience, 1,* 412–425.
Root, C., & Jenkins, J. (2005). Maternal appraisal styles, family risk status and anger biases of children. *Journal of Abnormal Child Psychology, 33,* 193–204.
Ruffman, T., Perner, J., Naito, M., Parkin, L., & Clements, W. (1998). Older (but not younger) siblings facilitate false belief understanding. *Developmental Psychology, 34,* 161–174.
Ruffman, T., Slade, L., & Crowe, E. (2002). The relation between children's and mothers' mental state language and theory-of-mind understanding. *Child Development, 73,* 734–751.
Ruffman, T., Taumoepeau, M., & Perkins, C. (2012). Statistical learning as a basis for social understanding in children. *British Journal of Developmental Psychology, 30,* 87–104.
Russell, J. (1997). *Autism as an Executive Disorder*. Oxford: Oxford University Press.
Sabbagh, M., Hopkins, S., Benson, J., & Flanagan, J. (2010). Conceptual change and preschoolers' theory of mind: Evidence from load-force adaptation. *Neural Networks, 23,* 1043–1050.
Salmon, K., Dadds, M., Allen, J., & Hawes, D. (2009). Can emotional language skills be taught during parent training for conduct problem children? *Child Psychiatry Human Development, 40,* 485–498.
Slaughter, V., & Gopnik, A. (1996). Conceptual coherence in the child's theory of mind: Training children to understand belief. *Child Development, 67,* 2967–2988.
Slaughter, V., Peterson, C., & MacKintosh, E. (2007). Mind what mother says: Narrative input and theory of mind in typical children and those on the autism spectrum. *Child Development, 78,* 839–858.
Taumoepeau, M., & Ruffman, T. (2008). Stepping stones to others' minds: Maternal talk relates to child mental state language and emotion understanding at 15, 24 and 33 months. *Child Development, 79,* 284–302.
Vygotsky, L. (1962). *Thought and Language*. Cambridge: MIT Press.
Wang, Q. (2008). On the cultural constitution of memory. *Memory, 16,* 305–317.
Wang, Q. (2012). Chinese socialization and emotion talk between mothers and children in native and immigrant Chinese families. *Asian American Journal of Psychology*. Epub ahead of print.
Wang, Q., & Fivush, R. (2005). Mother-child conversations of emotionally salient events: Exploring the functions of emotional reminiscing in European-American and Chinese families. *Social Development, 14,* 473–495.
Woolfe, T., Want, S., & Siegal, M. (2002). Signposts to development: Theory of mind in deaf children. *Child Development, 73,* 768–778.

Prof. Claire Hughes
Centre for Family Research, Department of Psychology
University of Cambridge, Free School Lane
Cambridge CB2 3RQ (UK)
E-Mail ch288@cam.ac.uk

Hansen Lagattuta K (ed): Children and Emotion. New Insights into Developmental Affective Sciences.
Contrib Hum Dev. Basel, Karger, 2014, vol 26, pp 106–118 (DOI: 10.1159/000354364)

The Mysterious Emotional Life of Little Red Riding Hood

Paul L. Harris[a] · Marc de Rosnay[b] · Samuel Ronfard[a]

[a]Department of Psychology, Harvard University, Cambridge, Mass., USA;
[b]School of Psychology, The University of Sydney, Sydney, N.S.W., Australia

Abstract

It is well-established that children realize around the age of 4 years that someone might approach a situation with a false belief about what it holds in store. Despite this insight, 4- and even 5-year-olds have difficulty in working out what the person will feel about the upcoming situation. They claim for example that even if Little Red Riding Hood mistakenly thinks there is only her grandmother waiting for her inside the cottage and that she knows nothing about the wolf, she will still feel afraid. We review a variety of experiments in which children display this gap between the grasp of a protagonist's emotion as compared to a protagonist's belief. We also describe new findings showing that children's attribution of emotion to a story character is a dynamic process. As the story character approaches an unexpected denouement, children's tendency to misattribute emotion intensifies. By implication, children's emotion attributions are not a fixed or static function of their current theory-of-mind. They fluctuate as the story unfolds.

When Little Red Riding Hood knocks on the door of her grandmother's cottage, does she feel afraid? For the adult who reads the classic story to a young child, the answer is straightforward. No, at that moment in the story, she doesn't feel afraid because she does not yet know what has happened to her grandmother. In fact, even when she goes into the cottage, she still does not fully understand the danger she is in. She is puzzled by what she sees – her grandmother looks strangely different. But she does not yet feel the intense fear that would be all too appropriate if she realized that a hungry wolf is in her grandmother's bed. This tension between the actual situation facing Little Red Riding Hood and her emotional reaction to that situation is obvious to the adult reader. But a solid body of findings shows that it is not obvious to young children. The dramatic irony of the story is lost upon them. They effectively jump the gun by attributing fear to Little Red Riding Hood even before she could know that there is something to be afraid of.

In this chapter, we discuss this fascinating and revealing lacuna in young children's understanding of emotion. We first describe some of the initial findings pointing to children's difficulty in understanding belief-based emotions. Second, we discuss an initially plausible explanation of that difficulty – the hypothesis that children fail to understand Little Red Riding Hood's mistaken beliefs and instead attribute her emotion to the situation that they know she faces. We will show that this goes part of the way toward an explanation but ultimately fails. Third, we review various studies that drive home the fact that there is a considerable lag between children's understanding of a protagonist's mistaken beliefs and their grasp of the emotions that flow from such beliefs. We also describe recent studies highlighting both the tenacity of children's misunderstanding as well as its lability. Finally, we propose an explanation for the overall pattern of findings.

A Nasty Surprise

Our first exploration of this topic was guided by the basic idea that at a certain point in development, children come to think about emotion like cognitive therapists. They come to acknowledge that emotional reactions depend not on the objective features of the situation that a person faces but on the person's appraisal of that situation. Even young preschoolers can make good use of a script-like analysis of what situations elicit particular emotions – for example, they attribute sadness to someone who has just lost a toy or happiness to someone who is about to get a treat [Borke, 1972]. Nevertheless, at some point they presumably appreciate that it is not the objective situation that causes emotion but a person's appraisal of that situation – be it mistaken or accurate – that is the critical determinant of what the person feels.

To examine this idea, we gave 4- and 6-year-olds a set of nasty surprise stories [Harris, Johnson, Hutton, Andrews & Cooke, 1989]. Children were first introduced to Mickey the Monkey, a toy monkey who was 'always playing tricks on the other animals'. Next, four other animals were presented and the desire of each animal for a particular food or drink was explained. For example, children were shown a toy bear and told: 'Bertie the Bear is very hungry and his favorite snack is Smarties (M&Ms)'. Bertie was then made to leave the scene to go for a walk. Next, the experimenter demonstrated how Mickey played a trick on Bertie. A Smarties box was introduced, Mickey was made to empty out all the Smarties and replace them with stones. The narrative continued: 'Mickey put the Smarties box with stones inside it on Bertie's table. Bertie came home and saw this Smarties box on his table.' Children were then asked three questions about Bertie's emotional reactions: (a) How does he feel when his Mom gives him a box of Smarties? (b) How does he feel when he first looks at the box on the table before he looks inside? (c) How will he feel when he has a look inside and finds that there are stones inside instead of Smarties? Comparable stories were told regarding three other victims of Mickey's mischief.

Across all four stories, both age groups were excellent at answering the first and third questions. They realized that the animals would normally feel happy at receiving a treat and sad at discovering the nasty surprise inside the container. As expected, the second question about the animal's initial reaction on seeing the gift from Mickey was much more challenging. With a few exceptions, the children answered according to one of two patterns. They either systematically claimed that the animal would be sad or they systematically claimed that the animal would be happy. The first pattern was common among 4-year-olds (55%) but infrequent among 6-year-olds (25%) whereas the second pattern was infrequent among 4-year-olds (35%) but frequent among 6-year-olds (70%).

Scrutiny of children's justifications reinforced this age change. Children who claimed that the animal would be sad typically explained that attribution by referring to the actual situation (e.g., 'there's no Smarties' or 'cos of the trick') whereas children who claimed that the animal would be happy often referred to the animal's desire for the treat that was apparently on offer (e.g., 'he likes Smarties') or ignorance of what was actually inside the container (e.g., 'cos she didn't see what's inside'). These results offered support for our initial hunch about the course of development. Younger children typically worked out what the animal was feeling by focusing on reality – the nasty trick that had been played by the mischievous monkey whereas older children were more likely to acknowledge the victim's naïve appraisal of reality.

A very similar pattern emerged in a second experiment in which we gave 4-, 5- and 6-year-olds either four nasty surprise stories – similar to those just described – or four pleasant surprise stories in which a now benign but nevertheless tricky Mickey again doctored the contents of a familiar container but introduced something desirable rather than undesirable. To take a concrete example, one of the tricked animals was Ellie the elephant. Children learned that Ellie liked only one kind of drink. Half the children were told that she liked only coke and the remaining children were told that she liked only milk. During her daily stroll in the jungle, Mickey tricked her by pouring the coke out of a coke can, replacing it with milk, and leaving the coke can on the table to await her return.

Children were asked how Ellie would feel on first spotting the coke can, and how she would feel after taking a sip. We reasoned that the second question was relatively straightforward: Children needed only to work out whether the actual contents – which she would discover on taking a sip – corresponded to Ellie's preferred drink – be it coke or milk. More specifically, as long as children realized that desires play a key role in determining emotional reactions, they would be expected to answer this question correctly – to appreciate that Ellie would get a nasty surprise if she preferred coke but a pleasant surprise if she preferred milk.

We expected the first question, by contrast, to prove more challenging. To answer correctly, children had to keep in mind Ellie's preferred drink – a preference that did not necessarily match their own. In addition they had to keep in mind whether or not the expected contents – coke, since it was a coke can – matched that preference. Effectively, children needed to coordinate their knowledge of Ellie's desire for a particular drink with an understanding of her mistaken presumption about the contents of the can.

Our expectations were borne out. Children in all three age groups performed very well on the second question. With few exceptions they answered correctly for all four stories. By implication, they had no difficulty in remembering the animals' individual preferences (e.g., for coke not milk – or vice versa) and in realizing whether a particular animal would end up having a nasty or pleasant surprise. Answers to the first question, by contrast, produced a marked age change. More than half of the 4-year-olds ignored the animals' mistaken belief and replied in terms of reality (i.e., what they knew to be inside the container). Only 19% managed to give correct replies on three or more stories (out of 4 trials). Among the 5- and 6-year-olds this percentage climbed to 44 and 75%, respectively. Using a much more liberal criterion – answering correctly on at least one trial – a similar change with age was observed. Thus, 38% of 4-year-olds, 63% of 5-year-olds and 88% of 6-year-olds were correct at least once.

The pattern of justification was very similar to that observed in the first experiment. Children tended to focus on either the reality of the situation or on the animal's mistaken appraisal of that reality with the latter pattern gradually displacing the former in the course of development. Taken together, these findings lent strong support to our expectation that children would increasingly realize that a person's emotion depends less on their actual circumstances than on their appraisal of those circumstances – even if the appraisal is ill-founded – and indeed will soon prove to be so. Setting these findings in the context of the story of Little Red Riding Hood, we would expect 4-year-olds to miss the protracted tension in the story – to assume prematurely that Little Red Riding Hood is afraid of the wolf.

On reflection, however, we realized that this straightforward developmental account overlooked something important. We shared our findings with Josef Perner who readily saw parallels with the classic false belief task that he and Heinz Wimmer had introduced some years earlier [Wimmer & Perner, 1983]. Still, he also pointed out that the parallel was less than exact. At the time, and indeed ever since [Wellman, Cross & Watson, 2001], the evidence shows that many 4-year-olds and most 5-year-olds do well on standard false belief tasks. By contrast, the success rate for our nasty and pleasant surprise tasks was a good deal poorer. For some mysterious reason, children found it hard to appreciate the impact of beliefs on emotion.

The puzzling nature of this lag did not fully sink in until it was dramatically highlighted in later experiments. But before describing those experiments it is worth underlining one initially appealing explanation of the lag. It might be argued that standard false belief tasks are relatively simple because they call only for a diagnosis of the protagonist's mistaken belief. By contrast, surprise tasks, whether nasty or pleasant, call for a diagnosis not just of the protagonist's mistaken belief but also a further inference about the protagonist's belief-based emotion. Perhaps it is this extra inferential step that creates the lag between the pattern of development for the standard false belief task and the pattern of development for the belief-based emotion tasks described above. However, this account ignores a crucial point. In most belief tasks [including Wimmer & Perner, 1983], children are not asked directly what the protagonist believes. Rather they are invited to work out what the protagonist will do – for example, where he or she will search – in the box or the cupboard. Alternatively, they are invited to work out whether a protagonist will say that there are pencils or M&Ms in a container [Gopnik & Astington, 1988]. In other words, the standard false belief tasks also call for an inferential step, whether it is from belief to action or from belief to utterance. So, the added difficulty of the emotion tasks cannot be due only to the addition of an inferential step. Of course, it might be the case that inferential steps are not equal in difficulty: The link between belief and emotion might be harder for children to understand than the link between belief and action or between belief and utterance. Still, that line of explanation – which we will return to later – implies that the problem has to do with the *nature* of the inference and not with making the inference per se.

What Does Little Red Riding Believe?

If there is indeed a developmental lag between children's diagnosis of a belief and their diagnosis of an ensuing belief-based emotion, we can predict that individual children will pass through a paradoxical phase in which they correctly diagnose the belief but incorrectly diagnose the emotion. Compelling evidence of this paradox was reported by Bradmetz and Schneider [1999]. Using the story of Little Red Riding Hood as a vehicle, they questioned children aged 3–6 years about her thoughts and feelings. For example, they asked, 'When Little Red Riding Hood goes into grandmother's house, does she think the wolf is in the bed or does she think the grandmother is in the bed?' and 'When Little Red Riding Hood goes into grandmother's house does she feel afraid? Why?'.

Almost half of the 3- and 4-year-olds answered both questions incorrectly, albeit coherently – they said that Little Red Riding Hood thought the wolf was in the bed and felt afraid. Conversely, nearly half of the 5- and 6-year-olds answered both questions correctly – they said that Little Red Riding Hood thought her grandmother was in the bed and did not feel afraid. The remaining children displayed the anticipated paradox – they diagnosed Little Red Riding Hood's belief correctly but not her emotion. They said that she thought it was her grandmother in the bed but then went on to claim that she felt afraid.

A similar pattern emerged in two follow-up studies by Bradmetz and Schneider [1999]. One was based on a story with a similar structure to Little Red Riding Hood involving a wolf that tricked a little goat. The other was closely modeled on a standard false belief task – Maxi, the main character, put his chocolate in a container and left the scene. In Maxi's absence, his brother ate most of the chocolate but put a small remaining piece in a different container. On Maxi's arrival at the door of his house, children were asked: 'Maxi is in front of the door, where will he look for his chocolate?' and 'When Maxi is in front of the door, is he happy?'.

In both studies, a décalage between replies to the two test questions was observed: Although children often replied incorrectly to both questions – or replied correctly to both questions – approximately half the children answered the belief question correctly and the emotion question incorrectly. The reverse pattern was never observed. By implication, a correct reply to the belief question is a necessary but not a sufficient condition for a correct reply to the emotion question.

Another experiment involving 6- to 8-year-olds further underlined children's persistent difficulty in appreciating the contradiction between their replies to the two questions. When children correctly said where Maxi would search, the interviewer posed the emotion question and then – depending on how children replied – offered a counter-suggestion. For example, children who incorrectly claimed that Maxi felt unhappy were asked whether he knew that his brother had eaten the chocolate. Children who correctly claimed that Maxi felt happy were reminded that his brother had eaten the chocolate. Then, in each case, the emotion question was repeated. These counter-suggestions had an impact but only in one direction. Among the children who had initially answered the emotion question correctly almost half changed their mind – reverting to an incorrect answer. By contrast, all the children who had initially answered the emotion question incorrectly – by claiming that Maxi was unhappy – clung to this incorrect answer.

Taken together, this series of experiments provides strong evidence for a paradoxical pattern of responding between the ages of 3 and 8 years. Children may appreciate the protagonist's mistaken belief but they do not necessarily work out the implications of that belief for what the protagonist feels – and even when they have done so, a counter-suggestion can easily unsettle them. To explain the gap between children's understanding of belief and their understanding of emotion, Bradmetz and Schneider [1999] proposed that emotional cues are vivid – their message has a high priority. Presumably, what these authors mean by this claim is that the affective implications of the situation facing the story character – whether or not he or she is aware of the situation – are strong and compelling for young children as they listen to the story. For example, as they listen to the story of Little Red Riding Hood they are likely to regard the wolf inside the grandmother's cottage as a strong and compelling cue for fear. That association between the wolf and the emotion of fear might be sufficiently rapid and vivid that children then attribute fear to Little Red Riding Hood even though they can work out that she was unaware of the presence of the wolf.

Indirect support for this line of interpretation can be gathered by thinking back to the influential findings of Zajonc [1980] on affective processing. He argued that the affective valence of a stimulus can be processed rapidly and efficiently. Indeed, in some cases, such processing can occur before the stimulus has even been recognized. For example, when presented with geometric shapes for brief intervals, adults did no better than chance at saying which stimuli they recognized as old versus new. Despite this absence of recognition, subjects expressed a preference for stimuli that they had seen before over those they had not.

On the other hand, when we take into account the full range of findings, an explanation for the belief-emotion gap in terms of the rapid and compelling nature of affective reactions begins to seem less plausible. Consider the experiment described earlier in which children listened to stories about animals with fairly idiosyncratic, and indeed narrow, preferences for a particular food or drink [Harris et al., 1989, experiment 2]. For example, Harry the Horse was described as liking only one kind of snack – either peanuts (for half the children) or chewing gum (for the other half). In either case, Mickey the monkey tricked Harry by replacing the contents of a peanuts packet with chewing gum. Can we maintain that chewing gum will immediately have negative implications for the children who have been told that Harry likes peanuts but positive implications for the children who have been told that he likes chewing gum? To the extent that children recognized that chewing gum has different implications for Harry depending on his desires, it would seem wrong to insist that it carries an automatic and inevitable affective message. We need to recognize that even younger children fine-tune the affective message depending on the particular, idiosyncratic desires of the protagonist.

To summarize the pattern of results so far, then, young children are oddly incoherent in their reasoning about mental states. On the one hand, they understand by 4 or 5 years of age that a protagonist may misconstrue reality – for example, by mistakenly thinking that there are Smarties in a Smarties box, that grandmother is in her bed, or that chocolate is in the same place as before. On the other hand, children of this age are prone to attribute emotion to that same protagonist on the basis of what they themselves know to be really the case, ignoring what the protagonist thinks to be the case. We have examined two initially plausible explanations and found them wanting. The proposal that emotion attributions are difficult because they call for some extra inferential step appears to be inadequate – standard tests of belief attributions also call for some extra inferential step – linking the belief to an action or utterance. Similarly, the proposal that emotion attributions might be disrupted by affectively charged cues that are rapidly processed sounds plausible for lurking wolves but less plausible for an unexpected packet of chewing gum that would disappoint one animal but please another. In the next sections, we discuss whether children show this lag on other belief-emotion problems as well as describe relations between performance and individual differences in language ability and input. Finally, we seek to offer a more adequate explanation of the pattern of results.

Beliefs, Emotion, and Language

Attachment theorists have suggested that children's understanding of emotion is likely to depend on the extent to which they can express, think about, and discuss their feelings in the context of a secure attachment relationship [Cassidy, 1994]. In an exploration of such individual differences, De Rosnay and Harris [2002] asked whether attachment security was linked to performance on different variants of the nasty surprise task and this offered an opportunity to ask a simple but important question. Do individual children perform in a consistent fashion across different variants of the task? In an initial examination of this question, children ranging from 3 to 6 years were given three different tasks. The dog-rabbit task was very similar to the nasty surprise tasks devised by Harris and his colleagues [Harris et al., 1989]. Children were introduced to Roger Rabbit and told that he likes Smarties and dislikes peanuts. Gromit the dog then played a trick on Roger by removing Smarties from a Smarties box, replacing them with peanuts, and leaving the box to await Roger's return.

A second task was quite different in both content and format. Children saw a short video clip showing a toddler left alone in a waiting room while her mother went to another room for an appointment. At a certain point, there was a knock at the door but to the toddler's disappointment, it was a stranger who came in rather than her mother. Children were asked how the toddler felt on first hearing the knock at the door. The rationale for this choice of content was that the video played on attachment-related themes, notably separation from the mother and a hoped-for reunion. Accordingly, it might be expected that secure children would be especially good at understanding the toddler's mistaken hope that his mother was returning.

The third task was similar to the second but more emotionally charged. Children saw a video clip showing a toddler left alone in a waiting room by his mother but in this case the toddler reacted to her departure with considerable distress. A knock at the door again proved misleading – and upsetting – because it was a stranger who entered rather than the mother.

Despite the variation among the three tasks with respect to the identity of the main protagonist, the nature of the protagonist's mistaken expectation, the degree of expressed emotion, and the format of the presentation, children proved to be quite stable in their performance on the key test questions in which they were asked to predict and explain how the protagonist felt (when seeing the Smarties box or when hearing the knock at the door). Thus, when performance on any two of the three tasks was compared, children tended to either pass both or fail both tasks. Indeed, performance on the Dog-Rabbit task and the more emotionally charged maternal separation task was highly concordant, with 44 of the total sample of 51 children (86%) either failing both or passing both. Note that these results cast further doubt on the explanation in terms of emotional vividness discussed earlier. That is to say, the prospect of disappointment would seem to be more compelling for the maternal separation video depicting a distressed toddler hearing a stranger's knock at the door compared to the prospect of disappointment in the case of Roger Rabbit. After all, he is simply getting peanuts (a snack that children might actually like) instead of getting Smarties. Yet, children responded similarly in each case.

Nevertheless there were considerable individual differences among the children in their overall performance – for example, some children as young as 3 years 11 months were able to identify the protagonist's 'mistaken' emotion and to explain it appropriately for one of the three tasks whereas some children as old as 5 years 10 months failed to answer these two questions for all three tasks. A regression analysis highlighted the important role of language ability (as measured by the BPVS, a measure of receptive vocabulary) and also – consistent with the earlier findings of Fonagy, Redfern and Charman [1997] – the role of attachment security, as measured by the Separation Anxiety Test [Klagsbrun & Bowlby, 1976], in which children are invited to discuss the feeling of a protagonist who is depicted as experiencing separation from one or both parents. Neither chronological age nor gender made a significant independent contribution to emotion understanding. By contrast, verbal mental age independently explained a considerable portion of the variance in emotion understanding (27.2%), and attachment security accounted for a smaller but significant portion (8.4%).

A follow-up analysis of these same children cast more light on their difficulties with the task and also on the facilitating role of language ability [de Rosnay, Pons, Harris & Morrell, 2004]. In line with the findings of Bradmetz and Schneider [1999], there was clear evidence that an understanding of false belief may be necessary for an understanding of belief-based emotion but is not sufficient. On each task, very few children answered the emotion question correctly and the belief question incorrectly. By contrast, a considerable proportion of the children gave the wrong answer to the emotion question – failing to realize that the protagonist would feel happy – but correctly attributed a mistaken belief to the protagonists. Thus, when asked about what Roger Rabbit thought was in the box or who the toddlers thought was knocking at the door, children managed to answer correctly. Furthermore, children's language ability proved to be a predictor both of correct replies to the false belief question and also of correct replies to the emotion question. Indeed, the relation between language and correct replies to the emotion question held up even when the contribution of language to performance on the false belief question was taken into account. Making this same point differently, it appears that language serves as a stepping-stone at two successive points. It first contributes to children's understanding of false belief and then it makes an additional, further contribution to their understanding of belief-based emotion [Harris, de Rosnay & Pons, 2005]. These findings are, of course, consistent with the more general point that has emerged repeatedly, namely that children's insight into a protagonist's false belief about a situation is no guarantee that they will proceed to a correct diagnosis of the emotion triggered by such a false belief.

To consolidate this pattern of findings, De Rosnay et al. [2004] conducted a further study in which they measured not just children's understanding of beliefs and belief-based emotions (using the Dog-Rabbit task and the emotionally charged maternal separation task) but also the nature of the language environment that children were exposed to. The experimenter invited mothers to describe their children (aged between 4.5 and 6 years) with an open-ended prompt ('Can you describe [child's name] for me?'). The frequency with which mothers talked about their children's mental life was assessed. As in the earlier studies, there was a sizeable group of children who correctly diagnosed the protagonist's mistaken belief but failed to attribute the emotion that would be appropriate given that mistaken belief. For example, in the maternal separation task, 33% displayed this pattern whereas only 9% showed the reverse pattern (i.e., correctly attributed the emotion but not the mistaken belief). As usual, those children who attributed the wrong emotion cited the emotion that would be likely given the actual situation facing the protagonist. However, the gap between emotion understanding and belief understanding was less marked among children whose mothers were more 'mind-minded' in that they often talked often about their child's mental life when describing them [Meins, Fernyhough, Russell & Clark-Carter, 1998]. More specifically, mothers whose descriptions of their child included proportionately more references to the child's thoughts and feelings rather than to the child's behavioral or physical attributes had children who answered correctly to both the belief and emotion questions.

Summarizing, children are fairly stable in their grasp of belief-based emotions. They show the same pattern of correct – or incorrect – attribution across a variety of tasks. Correct attribution of emotion is associated with language in two ways. Children with greater language ability and children with mothers who use more mental-state language make more correct attributions. Moreover, the contribution of language cannot be explained by its well-known association with an understanding of false belief [Astington & Baird, 2005]. The contribution to an understanding of emotion emerges even when prior allowance is made for a contribution to the understanding of false beliefs. This pattern of findings reinforces the conclusion set out earlier; the understanding of belief-based emotion calls for some insight or ability that goes beyond an understanding of false beliefs.

Understanding Our Own Emotions

The studies so far have focused on children's ability to figure out what someone else feels – whether it is Maxi, Little Red Riding Hood, Roger Rabbit or a toddler in a video. But we can also ask how far children are able to report their own emotions accurately, especially when those emotions are based on a misconstrual. Consider the following variant on another classic false belief task. Children are shown a familiar box of Smarties and asked to indicate how they feel about eating what's inside. Next, they are shown the contents – which turn out to be inedible beads rather than candy. The beads are then poured back into the box and children are asked what they initially thought was inside the box and also how they felt about eating it.

Depending on how we identify our emotions, two different outcomes seem feasible. Suppose that particular emotions such as happiness or sadness are natural kinds, each associated with a distinctive inner feeling, a particular pattern of physiological arousal, and a distinctive mode of expression via the face, voice and posture. Classic theories of emotions, rooted in Darwin's evolutionary approach, have long advocated such distinctive emotional states [Ekman, 1999; Ekman, Campos, Davidson & de Waal, 2003]. On this view, when first shown the Smarties box, children would be likely to identify their emotional state – for example, their emotion at the prospect of eating Smarties – based on its distinctive inner quality. Subsequently, when they are asked to think back to how they felt before learning the actual contents of the Smarties box, they should be able to remember that specific emotional state – just as they might remember other feeling states, such as a feeling of thirst or an itch in the neck.

However, suppose instead that there is an inextricable link between appraisal processes and emotional experience. More specifically, suppose that a given emotional experience is constructed on the basis of an appraisal of the situation that one faces [Lindquist & Barrett, 2008]. In that case, faced with a Smarties box and the prospect of eating the candy inside it, children might appraise the situation positively and judge themselves to be happy – not so much because of some identifiable inner glow of happiness but because they know that such a feeling is appropriate to the pleasant prospect of eating candy. On this view, it might be difficult for children to reconstruct their feelings about the prospect of Smarties, once that prospect is no longer in the offing. An accurate reconstruction of how they felt would call for: (a) an accurate retrieval of how they first viewed the Smarties box, and (b) an inference as to what they would have felt given that mistaken appraisal. But rather than engage in such a two-step accurate reconstructive process, children might instead take their current appraisal as a guide. Because they now view the box negatively – after all it contains only inedible beads – they may claim to have felt negatively even when first shown the box.

To compare these alternative accounts, Bender and his colleagues [Bender, Pons, Harris & de Rosnay, 2011] interviewed 5.5-year-olds and 7-year-olds. When presented with a nasty surprise along the lines just described, a considerable proportion of children especially in the older group displayed the by now familiar pattern. Although they correctly stated that they had initially thought there were Smarties in the box, they incorrectly stated that they had felt sad about eating the contents. Thus, even with respect to their own emotions, children were prone to report an emotion that was appropriate to what lay in store for them but inappropriate given their ignorance at the time. By implication, children did not report on their past emotion by delving into their memory and retrieving the record of some inner glow when they were first offered the Smarties box. Their report of their past emotion was contaminated by knowledge of what they discovered later – even if this knowledge did not contaminate their report of their past belief.

Overview and Interpretation

Summing up the pattern of findings, across a variety of different procedures and laboratories, young children around the age of 4 and 5 years can often do quite well in appreciating that someone who lacks the relevant perceptual access to a given situation may misconstrue that situation. Thus, children of this age realize that someone might think that a situation is rewarding or safe when, in fact, it is not. Despite this facility in understanding how a person – including themselves – might not know about what is in store for them, children frequently misattribute emotions to that person. They attribute emotions that make sense only in light of the impending situation. It is as if children look too far ahead, ignoring the fact that the person does not yet know what lies in the future. The likelihood of these 'premature' attributions varies from child to child. Two different language measures have been shown to account for some of this variation. Children with superior language ability and children whose mothers make more references to mental states are less prone to making such misplaced attributions of emotion.

As discussed earlier, it is tempting to explain these errors in terms of the extra inferential step required when imputing a belief-based emotion – as opposed to a belief per se. Yet there is no indication that children invariably have difficulty with such additional inferencing: They readily work out what someone will say or do on the basis of a false belief. Similarly, although it is plausible that the vivid emotional implications of an upcoming surprise – such as the presence of a wolf – are rapidly processed and highly salient, it is less plausible that the affective implications of the machinations carried out by Mickey the Monkey or Roger Rabbit (e.g., the replacement of Smarties by peanuts) are so highly salient, especially when the valence of those implications depends on the particular preferences of the victim (e.g., for Smarties over peanuts or vice versa).

However, it is possible to construct a more complex account that builds on these ideas while taking care of the aforementioned objections. We may suppose that children ordinarily appraise an imminent situation in light of their own ongoing goals and preferences. However, it is also plausible that when thinking about another person – whether it is a friend, a child in a video, or a story protagonist – children readily adopt a different appraisal strategy. They evaluate the situation that the person is facing in light that person's ongoing goals and preferences – not their own. Indeed, Repacholi and Gopnik [1997] showed that this flexibility emerges at an early age: having seen an adult express a preference for broccoli over crackers, toddlers who responded to the adult's request for food typically offered broccoli – even though the adult had not identified which particular food they were requesting.

So, when asked to say how a person feels, it is plausible that young preschoolers are able to attribute emotions based on a rapid appraisal of whether the situation that the person is facing matches that person's desires or not. Making the same point differently, an inhibitory process will be needed for that desire-based attribution process to be overridden. Knowing that the person is, in fact, unaware of the actual nature of the situation can, in principle, trigger such an inhibitory process but – as we have seen repeatedly – it may fail to do so. On this account, from 4 years of age and upward, children make progress in attributing emotion not in their ability to analyze what the person thinks, but in their ability to use the outcome of that analysis to override a powerful, desire-based analysis of the person's emotion.

This hypothesis implies that children will vary in the emotion that they attribute depending on whether the situation that the protagonist is approaching is a long way off – or imminent. When the situation is imminent, its positive and negative features – as appraised through the lens of the protagonist's desires – will be highly salient. Hence, the inhibitory process may not be effective enough to suppress an attribution of emotion based on its perceived valence for the protagonist. On the other hand, when the upcoming situation is more distant, the inhibitory process is more likely to succeed because the positive or negative features of the upcoming situation will be less salient.

We have recently tested this idea in a series of studies [Ronfard & Harris, 2013]. Children were reminded of the story of Little Red Riding Hood and then invited to consider her feelings as she made her way from her home toward her grandmother's cottage. More specifically, a figurine depicting Little Red Riding Hood was placed at four successive locations (at her own house, part way toward Grandmother's house, still closer to Grandmother's house and outside Grandmother's front door). Children were asked to say how Little Red Riding Hood felt at each successive location. In two experiments, a marked effect of distance was observed. Children were more prone to claim that little Red Riding Hood was afraid the closer she got to her destination. In a third experiment, children were asked about a protagonist who set off toward his own house, where unbeknownst to him, all his friends were waiting to play with him. A similar distance effect was observed but this time, it was misattributions of joy that became more frequent as the protagonist approached his destination.

An important implication of these findings is that children's attribution of emotion is not a fixed and direct function of their level of theory-of-mind understanding. In all three of the studies just described, individual children gave different answers depending on the distance of the protagonist from the upcoming surprise contrary to what we would expect if children's replies were entirely constrained by their theory-of-mind. The greater the immediacy of that surprise, the more children erred in their attributions. An important question for future research concerns the status of these fluctuating attributions. Should we insist that children 'really' do understand belief-based emotions as shown by their more accurate performance when the surprise is further away? On this view, the growing salience of the surprise masks what children really know about belief-based emotion. Alternatively, should we acknowledge that children do not actually understand belief-based emotions given their misattribution of emotion when a surprise is imminent?

The best way to resolve this dilemma is to think more carefully about how children make developmental progress between 4 and 6 years. According to one possibility – the inhibition account – progress simply calls for greater inhibitory control as indexed by standard tasks such as the day-night task [Carlson & Moses, 2001]. By implication, 4- and 5-year-olds do understand belief-based emotions but lack sufficient inhibitory control to set aside interference from the emotional implications of an upcoming surprise – and that shortfall is increasingly obvious the closer and more immediate the surprise. A different possibility is that development is primarily conceptual – it involves an increasingly firm grip on the idea that emotions flow from appraisal processes so that situations lying beyond a protagonist's awareness are not allowed to infect the emotion attribution process. According to this hypothesis, 4- and 5-year-olds might not genuinely understand belief-based emotions even when the protagonist is at far distances. The greater likelihood of correct attributions at more distant locations occurs primarily because the emotional implications of the upcoming surprise are less salient to children; therefore they cause less interference in making attributions to the protagonist.

To assess these two alternatives, it is helpful to think about the exact sequence and timing of the mental steps involved in attributing emotion. We may speculate that there are two different processes involved: a rapid, quasi-empathic process that specifies the emotional valence of an upcoming outcome in relation to the desires of a particular protagonist; and a slower, more conceptual and effortful process that first specifies which outcome the protagonist anticipates (especially in cases where the protagonist expects something different from the actual outcome) and then proceeds to specify the emotional valence of that anticipated outcome for the protagonist.

This model makes the following predictions: (a) children who mistakenly attribute fear to Little Red Riding Hood will do so quickly because they rely only on the faster process described above; (b) such mistaken attributions will be increasingly fast as the protagonist gets closer because the surprise will be increasingly salient to young children as they think about the movement and destination of the protagonist and notably his or her increasing proximity to the upcoming surprise; (c) the correct attribution of happiness to Little Red Riding Hood will be slower than incorrect attributions of fear because correct attributions of happiness call for the slower, reflective process described above, and, finally (d) the speed of such correct attributions will likely be slower at closer distances given the possibility of increased interference from the actual, upcoming situation in working out what exactly the protagonist anticipates.

How might we conceptualize developmental progress between 4 and 6 years of age in light of this model? One possibility is that both the faster, empathic process and the slower more conceptual process operate throughout that developmental period but that children become increasingly adroit at inhibiting and setting aside the output of the fast process and relying instead on the output of the slower process. Note that this corresponds to the assumptions of the inhibition account described above. If this account is correct, we can plausibly expect children to take more time to reply as they get older and shift from incorrect to correct replies. However, a second possibility is that the slower, more reflective process is only gradually put in place and becomes increasingly efficient and less effortful as children get older – effectively winning the race with the simpler empathic proves to supply an answer to the attribution question. This would be consistent with the second, more conceptually based account of development proposed above. On this hypothesis, we can plausibly expect that once children start to provide correct attributions (e.g., of no fear to Little Red Riding Hood), they will take increasingly less time to do so as compared to younger children because the slower, reflective process improves in efficiency.

In future research, we anticipate testing these various predictions by studying not just the accuracy or inaccuracy of children's attributions of emotion but also the speed with which they make those attributions. We also envisage examining the contribution of two other factors, one that we have already considered and one that we have touched on only in passing. If our analysis is correct, it should be feasible to alter the salience of the upcoming surprise for individual children. More specifically, depending on whether we ask children to attribute an emotion to the protagonist when he or she is at some distance from the upcoming surprise or alternatively, when it is imminent, the salience of that surprise should vary. In addition, if our emphasis on inhibitory control is correct, it is plausible that measures of individual differences in that ability will predict the ease or difficulty with which children inhibit their inclination to make attributions to the protagonist in light of the more rapidly, empathic process. We speculate that the pattern of performance elicited by variation in these two factors – relative distance from the surprise and inhibitory control may ultimately look quite similar. For example, children with superior inhibitory control would look similar to children tested when the protagonist is at some distance from the surprise and children with inferior inhibitory control would look similar to children tested when the protagonist is close to the surprise.

In conclusion, we are impressed by a nice paradox. Even if – as we have seen – children stumble in their attribution of belief-based emotions, they do make considerable progress in the space of 2 or 3 years. Developmental psychologists studying that progress, and seeking to understand it, are quite slow by comparison. After a quarter of a century of puzzlement there are still unanswered questions. Still, we like to think we are moving forward – even if we are not exactly sure what lies in store.

Acknowledgement

The authors gratefully acknowledge helpful feedback from Kristin Hansen Lagattuta and Henry Wellman.

References

Astington, J.W., & Baird, J.A. (Eds.). (2005). *Why language matters for theory of mind.* New York: Oxford University Press.

Bender, P.K., Pons, F., Harris, P.L., & de Rosnay, M. (2011). Do young children misunderstand their own emotions? *European Journal of Developmental Psychology, 8*, 331–348.

Borke, H. (1972). Interpersonal perceptions of young children: Egocentrism or empathy. *Developmental Psychology, 7*, 104–106.

Bradmetz, J., & Schneider, R. (1999). Is Little Red Riding Hood afraid of her grandmother? Cognitive vs. emotional response to a false belief. *British Journal of Developmental Psychology, 17*, 501–514.

Carlson, S.M., & Moses, L.J. (2001) Individual differences in inhibitory control and children's theory of mind. *Child Development, 72*, 1032–1053.

Cassidy, J. (1994). Emotion regulation: Influences of attachment relationships. In N. Fox (Ed.), The development of emotion regulation: Biological and behavioral considerations. *Monographs of the Society for Research in Child Development, 59*, 228–249.

De Rosnay, M., & Harris, P.L. (2002). Individual differences in children's understanding of emotion: The roles of attachment and language. *Attachment and Human Development, 4*, 39–54.

De Rosnay, M., Pons, F., Harris, P.L., & Morrell, J.M.B. (2004). A lag between understanding false belief and emotion attribution in young children: Relationships with linguistic ability and mothers' mental state language. *British Journal of Developmental Psychology, 22*, 197–218.

Ekman, P. (1999). Basic emotions. In T. Dalgliesh & T. Power (Eds.), *Handbook of cognition and emotion* (pp. 45–60). New York: Wiley.

Ekman, P., Campos, J.J., Davidson, R.J., & deWaal, F. (2003). *Emotions inside out: 130 Years after Darwin's the expression of the emotions in man and animals.* New York: New York Academy of Science.

Fonagy, P., Redfern, S., & Charman, T. (1997). The relationship between belief-desire reasoning and a projective measure of attachment security (SAT). *British Journal of Developmental Psychology, 15*, 51–61.

Gopnik, A., & Astington, J.W. (1988). Children's understanding of representational change and its relation to the understanding of false belief and the appearance-reality distinction. *Child Development, 59*, 26–37.

Harris, P.L., de Rosnay, M., & Pons, F. (2005). Language and children's understanding of mental states. *Current Directions in Psychological Science, 14*, 69–73.

Harris, P.L., Johnson, C.N., Hutton, D., Andrews, G., & Cooke, T. (1989). Young children's theory of mind and emotion. *Cognition and Emotion, 3*, 379–400.

Klagsbrun, M., & Bowlby, J. (1976). Responses to separation from parents: A clinical test for young children. *British Journal of Projective Psychology & Personality Study, 21*, 7–27.

Lindquist, K.A., & Barrett, L.F. (2008). Constructing emotion: The experience of fear as a constructive act. *Psychological Science, 19*, 893–903.

Meins, E., Fernyhough, C., Russell, J., & Clark-Carter, D. (1998). Security of attachment as a predictor of symbolic and mentalising abilities: A longitudinal study. *Social Development, 7*, 1–24.

Repacholi, B.M., & Gopnik, A. (1997). Early reasoning about desires: Evidence from 14- and 18-month-olds. *Developmental Psychology, 33*, 12–21.

Ronfard, S., & Harris, P.L. (2013). When will Little Red Riding Hood become scared? Children's attribution of mental states to a story character. *Developmental Psychology.*

Wellman, H.M., Cross, D., & Watson, J. (2001). Meta-analysis of theory-of-mind development: The truth about false belief. *Child Development, 72*, 655–684.

Wimmer, H., & Perner, J. (1983). Beliefs about beliefs: Representation and constraining function of wrong beliefs in young children's understanding of deception. *Cognition, 13*, 103–128.

Zajonc, R.B. (1980). Feeling and thinking: Preferences need no inferences. *American Psychologist, 35*, 151–175.

Paul L. Harris
Harvard Graduate School of Education
503A Larsen Hall, Appian Way 14
Cambridge, MA 02138 (USA)
E-Mail paul_harris@gse.harvard.edu

Author Index

Subject Index